Overview-Map Key

Raleigh (p. 24)

T0151163

Durham (p. 130)

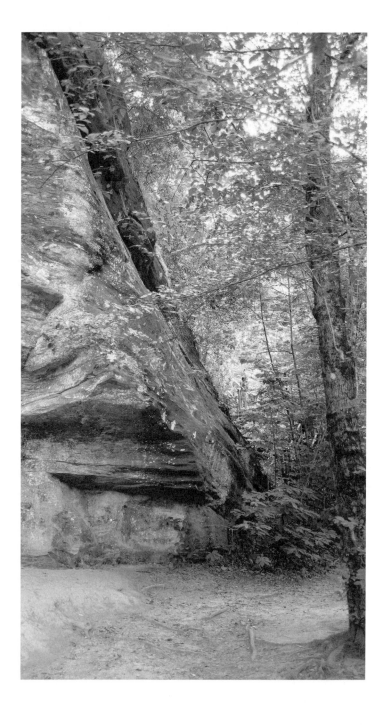

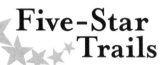

Five-Star Trails

Raleigh & Durham

Your Guide to the Area's Most Beautiful Hikes

Joshua Kinser

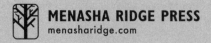

MENASHA RIDGE PRESS
menasharidge.com

Five-Star Trails: Raleigh & Durham

Copyright © 2013 by Joshua Kinser
All rights reserved
Published by Menasha Ridge Press
Distributed by Publishers Group West
Printed in the United States of America
First edition, first printing

Cover design and cartography by Scott McGrew
Front cover photo: Hike 30, Sarah P. Duke Gardens, see page 198
Back cover photo: Hike 23, Eno River State Park: Cox Mountain Trail, see page 157
Frontispiece: Hike 14, Raven Rock Loop, page 99
Text design by Annie Long
All photographs by Joshua Kinser except where noted
Indexing by Rich Carlson

Library of Congress Cataloging-in-Publication Data

Kinser, Joshua.
  Five-star trails Raleigh and Durham : your guide to the area's most beautiful hikes /
Joshua Kinser.
     p. cm.
  Includes index.
  ISBN 13: 978-0-89732-953-8 — ISBN 10: 0-89732-953-8
  e-ISBN: ISBN 978-0-89732-954-5
  1. Hiking—North Carolina—Raleigh Region—Guidebooks. 2. Hiking—North
Carolina—Durham Region—Guidebooks. 3. Trails—North Carolina—Raleigh
Region—Guidebooks. 4. Trails—North Carolina—Durham Region—Guidebooks.
5. Raleigh Region (N.C.)—Guidebooks. 6. Durham Region (N.C.)—Guidebooks.
I. Title.
  GV199.42.N662R3545 2013
  796.52097565—dc23

                            2012047136

Menasha Ridge Press
P.O. Box 43673
Birmingham, AL 35243
menasharidgepress.com

Disclaimer

This book is meant only as a guide to select trails in and
around Raleigh and Durham, North Carolina, and does not
guarantee hiker safety in any way—you hike at your own risk.
Neither Menasha Ridge Press nor Joshua Kinser is liable for
property loss or damage, personal injury, or death that result in any way from accessing
or hiking the trails described in the following pages. Please be especially cautious when
walking in potentially hazardous terrains with, for example, steep inclines or drop-
offs. Do not attempt to explore terrain that may be beyond your abilities. Please read
carefully the introduction to this book as well as further safety information from other
sources. Familiarize yourself with current weather reports and maps of the area you
plan to visit (in addition to the maps provided in this guidebook). Be cognizant of park
regulations and always follow them. *Do not take chances.*

Contents

Durham   130

Dedication

I would like to dedicate this book to the memory of Maritess "Tess" Demoret.

Acknowledgments

Thanks to all the trail crews and workers who have spent countless days in the dirt of the forest—chipping rock, cutting trees, cleaning trails and rivers, and constructing bridges—so that those of us who enjoy nature so much may have a path in which to explore it. Thank you, Jessica Nile, for all of your work and support. Thanks also to those who have advocated for the trails and greenways around Raleigh; they are some of the best in the country, and creating them is no easy task. Your work does not go unnoticed or unappreciated.

Also, thank you to Susan Haynes and Scott McGrew at Menasha Ridge Press for making this book possible.

—*Joshua Kinser*

Preface

For me, the Raleigh/Durham area used to be just a stop along my way to the Great Smoky Mountains. It was where I would swing by REI for a new camelback hose that always seemed to get moldy somehow, or to replace my worn hiking boots. I remember stopping by Raleigh on one trip and overhearing a woman say, "There's nothing to do in this town if you don't love the outdoors."

What's the opposite of a red flag? I guess a green flag is what went up in my mind. I decided that I should look into Raleigh a little bit more to see if this woman was right. I discovered she was—well, partially, at least. To be sure, there's a lot going on in Raleigh in general, but when it comes to the outdoors, and in particular hiking, Raleigh has definitely got it going on. Explore the surrounding cities of Durham and Chapel Hill, and what you find is a success-driven region with a passion and a deep commitment to enjoying, preserving, and sharing the rich natural environment of North Carolina's Piedmont and foothills.

Raleigh/Durham is nestled into one of North Carolina's sweetest spots. In the western part of the state, you are locked into a region of challenging mountains with difficult trails, climbing through a rugged terrain of rocks, steep gorges, exhausting ascents, and knee-grinding downhills. Go east of Raleigh and all you get is flat land. There are some beautiful forests, and the coastline and seascape are unimaginably beautiful, but it's still mostly flat farmlands. Raleigh/Durham is on the edge of the Piedmont, with the foothills to the west slowly rolling and building into the Appalachian ridge, and the valley of the eastern Piedmont thick with oak and pine forests, boardwalks running through bogs and wetlands, and grassy meadows filled with spring-blooming wildflowers. There is challenge in the hills, but no backbreaking mountains. There are easy routes through the Piedmont, but not the mind-numbing monotony and gradeless forests of the eastern flatlands. Venturing through all of these diverse settings are winding dirt-worn paths, paved running routes, and quiet, gravelly trails through leafy, shaded forests; along miles of snaking lakeshores; across grassy fields of city and rural parks; and amid the bustling business and historic districts of downtown Raleigh, Durham, and Chapel Hill.

If you're unsure where to start in your hiking explorations around Raleigh/Durham, then turn no further than page xii of this book, where you will find a list of recommended hikes divided into several different categories, so you can find exactly the experience you want. The trails in this book reflect the many different types of trails, terrain, and environments you can experience in the Raleigh/ Durham area. The featured routes come in a variety of lengths and difficulties, from a short and flat walk through a forest or around a small pond to an 8-mile adventure into the western foothills. These trails collectively capture the diversity of the landscape, the historical and natural highlights of the region, and the spirit of the area's impressive cities.

In these pages you will find long, challenging day hikes through the rolling forests of William B. Umstead State Park, snuggled between Raleigh and Durham; short journeys along the winding shores of Lake Jordan and Falls Lake; a walk through the artfully sculpted floral kaleidoscope that is Sarah P. Duke Gardens, in the heart of Duke University; a trek through downtown Durham, past the old tobacco warehouses and the Durham Bulls stadium; and a stroll along the leafy streets of Raleigh's historic Oakwood neighborhood, which features some of the best examples in the country of early-19th-century Victorian architecture. Die-hard wilderness adventurers and hard-core hikers have no need to worry, though. This is a book that mostly explores the wilderness and natural landscapes throughout this incredible and beautiful region.

It is my hope that *Five-Star Trails: Raleigh & Durham* contains the right trail for everyone, and that it reaches an audience interested in exploring all of the extremely diverse hiking and walking experiences that the Raleigh/Durham region has to offer. Please note, however, that this book is not a definitive collection of the absolute best day hikes in the region. Many additional miles of trails and paths wait to be explored—go out and discover them.

Recommended Hikes

Best Hikes for a Challenge

Best Hikes for Children

Best Hikes for Dogs

Best Easy Hikes

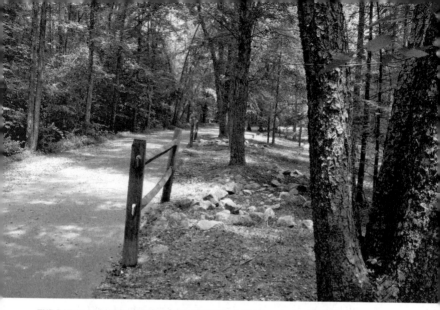

THE PATHS ARE IMPECCABLY MAINTAINED AT SHELLEY LAKE: SERTOMA PARK.

Best Hikes for Geology

Best Hikes for History

Best Hikes for Scenery

Best Hikes for Seclusion

Best Hikes for Wildflowers

Best Hikes for Wildlife

Introduction

About This Book

Five-Star Trails: Raleigh & Durham provides details, maps, elevation profiles, and photographs for 31 of the best hikes in this region. The Raleigh/Durham area is filled with incredible hiking routes that offer escapes to wilderness areas; walks through historic neighborhoods and business districts; and treks along greenway routes, through parks, and along the shores of the many lakes in this region. Raleigh/Durham lies within the rolling pine–oak forests of the eastern Piedmont, with the terrain becoming hillier to the west and the beginnings of the flat coastal plains emerging to the south and east.

While none of the hikes in this book merit five stars in every ratings category, some hikes get one, two, three, or four stars in one or more of them. A hike might earn inclusion in this book because the scenery is spectacular, while another hike with two-star scenery is selected because it's considered to be a five-star for kids. The star-rating system offers a simple and quick way to find the type of trail you are looking for.

Raleigh/Durham's Geographic Divisions

The hikes in this book have been divided into two geographic regions, each with its own particular attractions. You will find the best locations for trails in this region, which includes William B. Umstead State Park, Falls Lake State Recreation Area, Jordan Lake State Recreation Area, the Sarah P. Duke Gardens, and much more.

RALEIGH covers downtown, north to Durham Road, just past Cary to the east, south down to Lillington, and west to Knightdale. The walks in this section explore the highlights of the city that visitors and locals alike consider the best of Raleigh. The section includes a walk through the heart of Raleigh's downtown that explores Fayetteville

Street—the city's main artery through the financial and business district of downtown—and the City Market, a historic district that features a collection of shops and restaurants occupying classic red-brick storefronts, capturing the spirit of the traditional side of downtown Raleigh. This section also details a pleasant walk through one of the most popular historic neighborhoods in downtown Raleigh: Oakwood. Here you will find the homes of some of the early European settlers in Raleigh, as well as some of the finest examples of traditional Southern and Victorian architecture in the United States.

Other hikes in this section are centered on lakes. One explores Shelley Lake at Sertoma Park, about 5 miles north of downtown, while two other hikes venture along the southern portion of Falls Lake.

Historic Oak View County Park, a 27-acre farmstead site that can be explored along more than a mile of trails, is ideal for children. Along the mostly cobblestone- and brick-paved paths, you experience a historic barn, the main farmhouse, and a historic plank kitchen with an herb garden growing outside. Clemmons Educational State Forest offers another great trail for kids, with interpretive stations that teach children in a very fun way about the ecology, history, and geology of the forest.

At Historic Yates Mill County Park, you can walk a trail and discover the oldest gristmill still in operation in all of Wake County. Drive down to New Hill, North Carolina, and trek through the pine-and-oak forest along the perimeter of a peninsula that juts out into Harris Lake at Harris Lake County Park. Venture farther south to Raven Rock State Park and explore the intriguing rock formations along its wilderness trails.

Two trails explore the northern wilderness of William B. Umstead State Park. These unpaved paths follow along winding streams that cut through a rolling shady forest. Just east of Cary is Lake Johnson Park. This hike follows a paved path around the shore of Lake Johnson and over dramatic hills, with exceptional views of the lake nearly the entire time.

The **DURHAM** section takes you on a tour of the city center and surrounding attractions. For example, a guided tour of downtown's highlights features stops along "Black Wall Street," where the African American community established its main financial, banking, and investment hub. Take a walk to the Durham Bulls stadium, where the country's most famous minor-league baseball team plays. In this section you will also find a hike along the Al Buehler Cross Country Trail, nestled into Duke University's campus, as well as a tour of the Sarah P. Duke Gardens. If there is one place you want to visit on a trip to Durham, it is Duke Gardens, where you will discover an artfully landscaped world-class garden that hosts more than 300,000 visitors a year from all over the world.

North of Durham, venture on hikes into the foothills in parks such as Occoneechee Mountain State Natural Area and Eno River State Park. The hikes in this region offer a bit of challenge. The hilly terrain and hardwood forests along these routes provide a wilderness feel that can sometimes be lacking down in the Piedmont. A favorite trail in this area is the Cox Mountain Loop in Eno River State Park. Only 12 miles from Chapel Hill, this trail combines a challenging climb up Cox Mountain with a pleasant walk along the scenic Eno River for a trek that has the best of both worlds.

East of Durham you'll find a walk through the University of North Carolina at Chapel Hill campus. Along this walk you can explore all of the highlights of the campus, including the bell tower, Kenan Memorial Stadium, and the impressive and elegant Carolina Inn, as well as the restaurants, bars, and shops along Franklin Street. In this section you will also find a tour of the North Carolina Botanical Garden. Take a break from the hustle and bustle of Raleigh and head out to the Chapel Hill campus for a walk through the tranquil gardens in the heart of the university.

Jordan Lake is the highlight south of Durham. A 13,000-acre reservoir provides recreation for Raleigh/Durham residents, and the trails in this area give you a great introduction to the 32,000 acres of land that surround the enormous body of water. There are more than

22 miles of trails around Jordan. This book takes you to three impressive trails in three different recreation areas. Along these trails you will find top-notch picnic pavilions and sandy lakefront beaches that are perfect for sunning, relaxing, or a game of beach volleyball. Bring your swim trunks and your flip-flops with you. You might want them after you're done hiking these wonderful trails.

Falls Lake State Recreation Area, a 26,000-acre park, surrounds a 12,000-acre lake. Here, more than 20 miles of trails traverse six different recreation areas. Exceptional camping is offered in Falls Lake State Recreation Area during the summer, when most of the campgrounds are open. Turn your day hike into an overnight camping trip and continue to explore everything this area has to offer. You won't be disappointed.

How To Use This Guidebook

The following information walks you through this guidebook's organization to make it easy and convenient for planning great hikes.

Overview Map, Map Key, & Map Legend

The overview map on the inside front cover shows the primary trailheads for all 31 hikes. The numbers on the overview map pair with the map key on the facing page. A legend explaining the map symbols used throughout the book appears on the inside back cover.

Trail Maps

In addition to the overview map on the inside cover, a detailed map of each hike's route appears with its profile. On each of these maps, symbols indicate the trailhead, the complete route, significant features, facilities, and topographic landmarks such as creeks, overlooks, and peaks.

To produce the highly accurate maps in this book, I used a handheld GPS unit to gather data while hiking each route, then sent that data to Menasha Ridge Press's expert cartographers. Be aware, though, that your GPS device is no substitute for sound, sensible navigation that takes into account the conditions that you observe while hiking.

Further, despite the high quality of the maps in this guidebook, the publisher and myself strongly recommend that you always carry an additional map, such as the ones noted in each profile opener's "Maps" listing.

Elevation Profile

For trails with significant changes in elevation, the hike descriptions include this graphical element. Entries for fairly flat routes, such as a lake loop, do *not* display an elevation profile. Also, each entry's key information lists the elevation at the start of that specific route to its highest point.

For hike descriptions that include an elevation profile, this diagram represents the rises and falls of the trail as viewed from the side, over the complete distance (in miles) of that trail. On the diagram's vertical axis, or height scale, the number of feet indicated between each tick mark lets you visualize the climb. To avoid making flat hikes look steep and steep hikes appear flat, varying height scales provide an accurate image of each hike's climbing challenge.

The Hike Profile

Each profile opens with the hike's star ratings, GPS trailhead coordinates, and other key at-a-glance information—from the trail's distance and configuration to contacts for local information. Each profile also includes a map (see "Trail Maps"). The main text for each profile includes four sections: Overview, Route Details, Nearby Attractions, and Directions (for driving to the trailhead area).

Star Ratings

Five-Star Trails is the title of a Menasha Ridge Press guidebook series geared to specific cities across the United States, such as this one for Raleigh/Durham. Following is the explanation for the rating system of one to five stars in each of the five categories for each hike.

FOR SCENERY:

★ ★ ★ ★ ★   Unique, picturesque panoramas

★ ★ ★ ★   Diverse vistas

★ ★ ★   Pleasant views

★ ★   Unchanging landscape

★   Not selected for scenery

FOR TRAIL CONDITION:

★ ★ ★ ★ ★   Consistently well maintained

★ ★ ★ ★   Stable, with no surprises

★ ★ ★   Average terrain to negotiate

★ ★   Inconsistent, with good and poor areas

★   Rocky, overgrown, or often muddy

FOR CHILDREN:

★ ★ ★ ★ ★   Babes in strollers are welcome

★ ★ ★ ★   Fun for any kid past the toddler stage

★ ★ ★   Good for young hikers with proven stamina

★ ★   Not enjoyable for children

★   Not advisable for children

FOR DIFFICULTY:

★ ★ ★ ★ ★   Grueling

★ ★ ★ ★   Strenuous

★ ★ ★   Moderate—won't beat you up, but you'll know you've been hiking

★ ★   Easy with patches of moderation

★   Good for a relaxing stroll

FOR SOLITUDE:

★ ★ ★ ★ ★   Positively tranquil

★ ★ ★ ★   Spurts of isolation

★ ★ ★   Moderately secluded

★ ★   Crowded on weekends and holidays

★   Steady stream of individuals and/or groups

GPS TRAILHEAD COORDINATES

As noted in "Trail Maps," on page 4, I used a handheld GPS unit to obtain geographic data and sent the information to the cartographers at Menasha Ridge. In the opener for each hike profile, the coordinates—the intersection of latitude (north) and longitude (west)—will orient you from the trailhead. In some cases, you can drive within viewing distance of a trailhead. Other hiking routes require a short walk to the trailhead from a parking area.

This guidebook uses the degree–decimal minute format for expressing GPS coordinates. The latitude–longitude grid system is likely quite familiar to you, but here's a refresher, pertinent to visualizing the coordinates:

Imaginary lines of latitude—called *parallels* and approximately 69 miles apart from each other—run horizontally around the globe. The equator is established to be 0°, and each parallel is indicated by degrees from the equator: up to 90°N at the North Pole, and down to 90°S at the South Pole.

Imaginary lines of longitude—called *meridians*—run perpendicular to lines of latitude and are likewise indicated by degrees. Starting from 0° at the Prime Meridian in Greenwich, England, they continue to the east and west until they meet 180° later at the International Date Line in the Pacific Ocean. At the equator, longitude lines also are approximately 69 miles apart, but that distance narrows as the meridians converge toward the North and South Poles.

To convert GPS coordinates given in degrees, minutes, and seconds to degrees–decimal minutes, the seconds are divided by 60. For more on GPS technology, visit **usgs.gov.**

DISTANCE & CONFIGURATION

Distance indicates the length of the hike from start to finish, either round-trip or one-way depending on the trail configuration. If the hike description includes options to shorten or extend the hike, those distances will also be factored here. *Configuration* defines the type of route—for example, an out-and-back (which takes you in and out the same way), a figure eight, a loop, or a balloon.

HIKING TIME

Two miles per hour is a general rule of thumb for hiking the trails in this book, depending on the terrain and whether you have children with you. That pace typically allows time for taking photos, for dawdling and admiring views, and for alternating stretches of hills and descents. When deciding whether or not to follow a particular trail in this guidebook, consider your own pace, the weather, your general physical condition, and your energy level on a given day.

HIGHLIGHTS

This section lists features that draw hikers to the trail: waterfalls, historic sites, and the like.

ELEVATION

In each hikes's key information, you will see the elevation (in feet) at the trailhead and another figure for the peak height you will reach on the trail. For routes that involve significant ascents and descents, the hike profile also includes an elevation diagram (see page 5).

ACCESS

Fees or permits required to hike the trail are detailed here—and noted if there are none. Trail-access hours are also shown here.

MAPS

Resources for maps, in addition to those in this guidebook, are listed here. (As previously noted, the publisher and author recommend that you carry more than one map—and that you consult those maps before heading out on the trail to resolve any confusion or discrepancy.)

FACILITIES

Includes restrooms, phones, water, picnic tables, and other basics at or near the trailhead.

WHEELCHAIR ACCESS

Notes paved sections or other areas where persons with disabilities can safely use a wheelchair.

COMMENTS

Here you'll find assorted nuggets of information, such as whether or not dogs are allowed on the trails.

CONTACTS

Listed here are phone numbers and website addresses for checking trail conditions and gleaning other day-to-day information.

Overview, Route Details, Nearby Attractions, & Directions

These four elements provide the main text about the hike. "Overview" gives you a quick summary of what to expect on that trail; the "Route Details" guide you on the hike, start to finish; "Nearby Attractions" suggests appealing area sites, such as restaurants, museums, and other trails. "Directions" will get you to the trailhead from a well-known road or highway.

Weather

In Raleigh and Durham, you can experience all four seasons, but the summer is long and the spring and fall are fairly short. So be prepared for hot temperatures much of the year. Enjoy the variations, but always give careful consideration to weather and prepare accordingly.

Summers can be brutally hot. This is the time to get out of the sweltering heat of the city and head to the shady forests and trails that follow along waterways. Destinations farther out are always going to be a few degrees cooler than the city, so don't let the heat stop you from exploring. Plan to hike during the morning and evening, and make sure to bring plenty of water. Summer can also bring afternoon thunderstorms and dangerous lightning storms to the region, so this is yet another reason to consider hiking in the morning or evening during the summer.

Spring and fall are short around Raleigh and Durham, but these seasons are absolutely the best times for hiking anywhere in and around the city. Spring weather can be volatile and unpredictable: a warm and sunny day can turn into a cool and rainy one in a matter of hours. Visitors flock to the most popular trails in the fall, as the leaves begin to turn and display their colors. During these peak seasons, you should consider hiking early in the morning or during weekdays to avoid crowds.

Winter in this part of North Carolina is comparatively mild, with temperatures only occasionally dropping below freezing. Therefore, it's rarely too cold to hike in this region if you dress for the weather. If solitude is what you see, winter is a great season to hit the trails around the Raleigh and Durham region. In the winter, plan accordingly in terms of attire and, very important, in terms of time: winter daylight hours are short, especially if you are hiking in forested areas.

The following chart lists average temperatures and precipitation by month for the Raleigh/Durham region. For each month, "Hi Temp" is the average daytime high, "Lo Temp" is the average nighttime low, and "Rain or Snow" is the average precipitation.

RALEIGH			
MONTH	HI TEMP	LO TEMP	RAIN or SNOW
January	51°F	32°F	4.5"
February	56°F	34°F	3.6"
March	64°F	41°F	4.5"
April	73°F	48°F	3.0"
May	79°F	57°F	3.9"
June	86°F	65°F	4.0"
July	89°F	69°F	4.5"
August	87°F	68°F	4.2"
September	82°F	62°F	4.4"
October	72°F	50°F	3.6"
November	63°F	42°F	3.2"
December	54°F	35°F	3.2"

DURHAM			
MONTH	HI TEMP	LO TEMP	RAIN or SNOW
January	49°F	28°F	4.5"
February	53°F	29°F	3.7"
March	62°F	37°F	4.7"
April	71°F	46°F	3.4"
May	79°F	56°F	4.6"
June	85°F	65°F	4.0"
July	89°F	70°F	3.9"
August	87°F	68°F	4.4"
September	81°F	60°F	4.4"
October	71°F	47°F	3.7"
November	62°F	37°F	3.4"
December	53°F	30°F	3.4"

Water

How much is enough? Well, one simple physiological fact should convince you to err on the side of excess when deciding how much water to pack: a hiker walking steadily in 90° heat needs approximately 10 quarts of fluid per day. That's 2.5 gallons. A good rule of thumb is to hydrate prior to your hike, carry (and drink) 6 ounces of water for every mile you plan to hike, and hydrate again after the hike. For most people, the pleasures of hiking make carrying water a relatively minor price to pay to remain safe and healthy. So pack more water than you anticipate needing even for short hikes.

If you find yourself tempted to drink "found water," proceed with extreme caution. Many ponds and lakes you'll encounter are fairly stagnant, and the water tastes terrible. Drinking such water presents inherent risks for thirsty trekkers. Giardia parasites contaminate many water sources and cause the dreaded intestinal ailment giardiasis, which can last for weeks after onset. For more information, visit the Centers for Disease Control and Prevention website: **cdc.gov/parasites/giardia.**

In any case, effective treatment is essential before you drink from any water source along the trail. Boiling water for 2–3 minutes is always a safe measure for camping, but day hikers can consider iodine tablets, approved chemical mixes, filtration units rated for giardia, and UV filtration. Some of these methods (for example, filtration with an added carbon filter) remove bad tastes typical in stagnant water, while others add their own taste. As a precaution, carry a means of water purification to help in a pinch and if you realize you have underestimated your consumption needs.

Clothing

Weather, unexpected trail conditions, fatigue, extended hiking duration, and wrong turns can individually or collectively turn a great outing into a very uncomfortable one at best—and a life-threatening one at worst. Thus, proper attire plays a key role in staying comfortable and, sometimes, in staying alive. Here are some helpful guidelines:

★ Choose silk, wool, or synthetics for maximum comfort in all of your hiking attire—from hats to socks and in-between. Cotton is fine if the weather remains dry and stable, but you won't be happy if that material gets wet.

★ Always wear a hat, or at least tuck one into your day pack or hitch it to your belt. Hats offer all-weather sun and wind protection as well as warmth if it turns cold.

★ Be ready to layer up or down as the day progresses and the mercury rises or falls. Today's outdoor wear makes layering easy, with such designs as jackets that convert to vests and zip-off or button-up legs.

★ Wear hiking boots or sturdy hiking sandals with toe protection. Flip-flopping along a paved urban greenway is one thing, but never hike a trail in open sandals or casual sneakers. Your bones and arches need support, and your skin needs protection.

★ Pair that footwear with good socks! If you prefer not to sheathe your feet when wearing hiking sandals, tuck the socks into your day pack;

you may need them if the weather plummets or if you hit rocky turf and pebbles begin to irritate your feet. And in an emergency, if you've lost your gloves, you can adapt the socks into mittens.

★ Don't leave rainwear behind, even if the day dawns clear and sunny. Tuck into your day pack, or tie around your waist, a jacket that is breathable and either water-resistant or waterproof. Investigate different choices at your local outdoors retailer.

★ If you're a frequent hiker, ideally you'll have more than one rainwear weight, material, and style in your closet to protect you in all seasons in your regional climate and hiking microclimates.

Essential Gear

Today you can buy outdoor vests that have up to 20 pockets shaped and sized to carry everything from toothpicks to binoculars. Or, if you don't aspire to feel like a burro, you can neatly stow all of these items in your day pack or backpack. The following list showcases never-hike-without-them items—in alphabetical order, as all are important:

★ *Extra food:* trail mix, granola bars, or other high-energy snacks.

★ *Extra clothes:* raingear, a change of socks, and depending on the season, a warm hat and gloves.

★ *Flashlight or headlamp* with extra bulb and batteries.

★ *Insect repellent.* For some areas and seasons, this is vital.

★ *Maps and a high-quality compass.* Even if you know the terrain from previous hikes, don't leave home without these tools. And, as previously noted, bring maps in addition to those in this guidebook, and consult your maps prior to the hike. If you're GPS-savvy, bring that device, too, but don't rely on it as your sole navigational tool—battery life is limited, after all—and be sure to check its accuracy against that of your maps and compass.

★ *Pocketknife and/or multitool.*

★ *Sunscreen.* Check the expiration date on the tube or bottle.

★ *Water.* As we've emphasized more than once, bring more than you think you'll drink. Depending on your destination, you may want to bring a container and iodine or a filter for purifying water in case you run out.

★ *Whistle.* It could become your best friend in an emergency.

★ *Windproof matches and/or a lighter,* as well as a fire starter.

First-Aid Kit

In addition to the items above, those below may appear overwhelming for a day hike. But any paramedic will tell you that the products listed here—again, in alphabetical order, because all are important—are just the basics. The reality of hiking is that you can be out for a week of backpacking and acquire only a mosquito bite. Or you can hike for an hour, slip, and suffer a bleeding abrasion or broken bone. Fortunately, these listed items will collapse into a very small space. You also may purchase convenient, prepackaged kits at your pharmacy or on the Internet.

★ Ace bandages or Spenco joint wraps

★ Adhesive bandages

★ Antibiotic ointment (Neosporin or the generic equivalent)

★ Athletic tape

★ Benadryl or the generic equivalent, diphenhydramine (in case of allergic reactions)

★ Blister kit (such as Moleskin or Spenco 2nd Skin)

★ Butterfly-closure bandages

★ Epinephrine in a prefilled syringe (typically by prescription only, and for people known to have severe allergic reactions to hiking mishaps such as bee stings)

★ Gauze (one roll and a half-dozen 4-by-4-inch pads)

★ Hydrogen peroxide or iodine

★ Ibuprofen or acetaminophen

Note: Consider your intended terrain and the number of hikers in your party before you exclude any article listed above. A botanical-garden stroll may not inspire you to carry a complete kit, but anything beyond that warrants precaution. When hiking alone, you should always be prepared for a medical need. And if you're a twosome or with a group, one or more people in your party should be equipped with first-aid material.

General Safety

The following tips may have the familiar ring of Mom's voice as you take note of them.

★ *Always let someone know where you'll be hiking and how long you expect to be gone.* It's a good idea to give that person a copy of your route, particularly if you're headed into any isolated area. Let him or her know when you return.

★ *Always sign in and out of any trail registers provided.* Don't hesitate to comment on the trail condition if space is provided; that's your opportunity to alert others to any problems you encounter.

★ *Don't count on a cell phone for your safety.* Reception may be spotty or nonexistent on the trail, even on an urban walk—especially one embraced by towering trees or buildings.

★ *Always carry food and water, even for a short hike.* And bring more water than you think you'll need. (We can't emphasize this enough!)

★ *Ask questions.* Public-land employees are on hand to help. It's a lot easier to solicit advice before a problem occurs, and it will help you avoid a mishap away from civilization when it's too late to amend an error.

★ *Stay on designated trails.* Even on the most clearly marked trails, you usually reach a point where you have to stop and consider in which direction to head. If you become disoriented, don't panic. As soon as you think you may be off-track, stop, assess your current direction, and then retrace your steps to the point where you went astray. Using a map, a compass, and this book, and keeping in mind what you've passed thus far, reorient yourself, and trust your judgment on which way to continue. If you become absolutely unsure of how to continue, return to your vehicle the way you came in. Should you become completely lost and have no idea how to find the trailhead, remaining in place along the trail and waiting for help is most often the best option for adults, and always the best option for children.

★ *Always carry a whistle,* another precaution that we can't over-emphasize. It may become a lifesaver if you get lost or hurt.

★ *Be especially careful when crossing streams.* Whether you're fording the stream or crossing on a log, make every step count. If you have any doubt about maintaining your balance on a log, ford the stream instead: use a trekking pole or stout stick for balance and *face upstream as you cross.* If a stream seems too deep to ford, turn back. Whatever is on the other side isn't worth risking your life for.

★ *Be careful at overlooks.* While these areas may provide spectacular views, they are potentially hazardous. Stay back from the edge of outcrops, and make absolutely sure of your footing—a misstep can mean a nasty and possibly fatal fall.

★ *Standing dead trees and storm-damaged living trees pose a significant hazard to hikers.* These trees may have loose or broken limbs that could fall at any time. While walking beneath trees, and when choosing a spot to rest or enjoy your snack, look up!

★ *Know the symptoms of subnormal body temperature, or hypothermia.* Shivering and forgetfulness are the two most common indicators of this stealthy killer. Hypothermia can occur at any elevation, even in the summer, especially when the hiker is wearing lightweight cotton clothing. If symptoms develop, get to shelter, hot liquids, and dry clothes ASAP.

★ *Likewise, know the symptoms of heat exhaustion, or hyperthermia.* Lightheadedness and loss of energy are the first two indicators. If you feel these symptoms, find some shade, drink your water, remove as many layers of clothing as practical, and stay put until you cool down. Marching through heat exhaustion leads to heatstroke—which can be deadly. If you should be sweating and you're not, that's the signature warning sign. Your hike is over at that point: heatstroke is a life-threatening condition that can cause seizures, convulsions, and eventually death. If you or a companion reaches that point, do whatever you can to cool down, and seek medical attention immediately.

★ *Most importantly, take along your brain.* A cool, calculating mind is the single-most important asset on the trail. It allows you to think before you act.

★ *In summary:* Plan ahead. Watch your step. Avoid accidents before they happen. Enjoy a rewarding and relaxing hike.

Watchwords for Flora & Fauna

Hikers should remain aware of the following concerns regarding plant life and wildlife, described in alphabetical order.

Black Bears

Though attacks by black bears are uncommon, they have occurred around the Raleigh/Durham area. The highest concentration of black bears will most likely be found north of Raleigh/Durham in the more mountainous areas, but you may encounter a black bear in any of the natural areas in this region.

If you come upon a bear while hiking, remain calm and resist the urge to run. Make loud noises to scare off the bear and back away slowly. In primitive and remote areas, assume bears are present; in more-developed sites, check on the current bear situation prior to hiking. Most encounters are food-related, as bears have an exceptional sense of smell and not particularly discriminating tastes. While this is of greater concern to backpackers and campers, on a day hike, you may plan a lunchtime picnic or will munch on an energy bar or other snack from time to time. So remain aware and alert.

Black Flies

Though certainly a maddening annoyance, a black fly will at worst cause an itchy welt. They are most active from mid-May into June, during the day, and especially before thunderstorms, as well as during the morning and evening. Insect repellent has some effect, though the only way to keep out of their swarming midst is to keep moving.

Mosquitoes

Ward off these pests with insect repellent and/or repellent-impregnated clothing. In some areas, mosquitoes are known to carry the West Nile virus, so take extra care to avoid their bites.

Poison Ivy, Oak, & Sumac

Recognizing and avoiding poison ivy, oak, and sumac are the most effective ways to prevent the painful, itchy rashes associated with these plants. Poison ivy occurs as a vine or groundcover, three leaflets to a leaf; poison oak occurs as either a vine or shrub, also with three leaflets; and poison sumac flourishes in swampland, each leaf having 7–13 leaflets. Urushiol, the oil in the sap of these plants, is responsible for the rash. Within 14 hours of exposure, raised lines and/or blisters will appear on the affected area, accompanied by a terrible itch. Refrain from scratching, because bacteria under your fingernails can cause an infection.

Wash and dry the affected area thoroughly, applying calamine lotion to help dry out the rash. If the itching or blistering is severe, seek medical attention. To keep from spreading the misery to someone else, wash not only any exposed parts of your body but also any oil-contaminated clothes, hiking gear, and pets. Again, long pants and a long-sleeved shirt may offer the best protection.

Snakes

Rattlesnakes, cottonmouths, copperheads, and corals are among the most common venomous snakes in the United States, and their hibernation season is typically October–April. But despite their fearsome reputation, rattlesnakes like to bask in the sun and won't bite unless threatened.

In the region described in this book, you will possibly encounter rattlesnakes, copperheads, and water moccasins. However, the snakes you most likely will see while hiking will be nonvenomous species and subspecies. The best rule is to leave all snakes alone, give them a wide berth as you hike past, and make sure any hiking companions (including dogs) do the same.

When hiking, stick to well-used trails, and wear over-the-ankle boots and loose-fitting long pants. Do not step or put your hands beyond your range of detailed visibility, and avoid wandering around in the dark. Step *onto* logs and rocks, never *over* them, and be especially careful when climbing rocks. Always avoid walking through dense brush or willow thickets.

Ticks

These arachnids are often found on brush and tall grass, where they seem to be waiting to hitch a ride on warm-blooded passersby. Adult ticks are most active April–May and again October–November. The black-legged (deer) tick is the primary carrier of Lyme disease.

A few precautions: Wear light-colored clothing, which will make it easy for you to spot ticks before they migrate to your skin. After hiking, inspect your hair, the back of your neck, your armpits, and your socks. During your posthike shower, take a moment to do a more complete body check. To remove a tick that is already embedded, use tweezers made just for this purpose. Treat the bite with disinfectant solution.

Hunting

A number of rules, regulations, and licenses govern the various hunting types and related seasons. Though no problems generally arise, hikers may wish to forgo their trips during the big-game seasons, when the woods suddenly seem filled with orange and camouflage. Hunting season in the Raleigh/Durham area lasts September 8–January 1.

Regulations

Each state generally has a unique set of regulations that apply to the use of its parks and other public lands. Below you will find many of the rules that are most important to know when visiting these areas. For more information, visit **ncparks.gov.**

★ Pets must be on a leash no longer than 6 feet at all times and must not be left unattended. Campers must confine pets to enclosed vehicles or tents during the park's quiet hours, and pets are not allowed in bathhouses, changing areas, rinsing stations, swimming areas, restrooms, visitor centers, or rental boats. Exceptions are service animals and authorized search-and-rescue dogs.

★ North Carolina state parks are wildlife preserves. The removal, destruction, or injury of any tree, flower, artifact, fern, shrub, rock, or other plant or mineral in any park is prohibited unless with an approved collection permit for scientific or educational purposes.

★ The hunting, trapping, pursuing, shooting, injuring, killing, molesting, feeding, or baiting of any bird or animal is prohibited.

★ In parks where boating and fishing are allowed during park hours, such activities are regulated by all applicable North Carolina laws and regulations, including those regarding fishing licenses, boat registration, and safety requirements.

★ For your safety and protection, please stay on designated trails and hiking areas. Also, many rare plants live on thin soils and wet rocks and are vulnerable to damage from climbing, trampling, and scraping.

Camping

★ In North Carolina, it is lawful to camp anywhere in a national forest unless it is otherwise posted. In state parks and national parks, the following are prohibited: alcohol, the possession or use of fireworks, cap pistols, air guns, bows and arrows, slingshots, or lethal missiles of any kind. To possess a handgun within a state or national park, you must have a concealed-handgun permit, and regardless, firearms are not allowed in any park offices or visitor centers.

★ As a courtesy to other campers, please observe the campground quiet hours, typically 10 p.m.–7 a.m. In any park or recreation area, sounds that annoy, disturb, or frighten park visitors are prohibited at all times.

★ Camping is allowed in designated areas by permit only. In most cases, campers register with a ranger on-site or at an on-site registration box. Fires are permitted only in designated areas and must be tended at all times. Gathering firewood is generally prohibited but may be allowed in some parks.

Litter

Littering is illegal in North Carolina.

★ To help maintain a clean and safe environment for park visitors and wildlife, place trash in proper containers. Wildlife may mistake plastic bags for food and may become entangled in discarded fishing line or other types of litter.

★ Burying trash is prohibited. Shifting winds and other types of weather may expose trash and endanger wildlife and the environment.

★ State law requires aluminum cans to be placed in recycling containers where available.

Business and Special Activities

Conducting commercial business or certain organized activities in North Carolina state parks is allowed only with a special-activity permit. Photography or video production for commercial purposes is prohibited unless you have a film permit.

State parks allow for many special recreational activities, such as bicycling events, marathons, photo tours, kite-flying contests, club meetings, and so on. However, all such events require a special-activity permit ($35). The permit application can be downloaded from the "Forms & Permits" link on the individual park pages at **ncparks.gov** or may be obtained from park offices.

Vehicles and Bicycles

★ North Carolina motor-vehicle and traffic laws apply in all state parks. Unlicensed motor vehicles—including golf carts, unregistered motorcycles, snowmobiles, utility vehicles, minibikes, and all-terrain vehicles—are prohibited.

★ Unlicensed drivers may not operate motor vehicles on park roads.

★ Motorized vehicles are permitted only in designated areas and not permitted on park trails.

★ All vehicles left in the park after posted park hours must be registered.

★ No carts, carriages, or other horse-drawn apparatus are permitted on park trails.

★ In all parks, bicycles are permitted only on those trails or other park areas specifically designated for their use.

★ Bicycle riders under age 16 must wear a helmet.

★ Bicycle passengers who weigh less than 40 pounds or who are less than 40 inches tall must be seated in a separate restraining seat. All other bicycle riders must be seated on saddle seats. Persons who are unable to maintain an erect seated position cannot be bicycle passengers.

Trail Etiquette

Always treat trails, wildlife, and fellow hikers with respect. Here are some reminders.

★ Plan ahead in order to be self-sufficient at all times. For example, carry necessary supplies for changes in weather or other conditions.

★ Hike on open trails only.

★ In seasons or construction areas where road or trail closures may be a possibility, use the website addresses or phone numbers shown in the "Contacts" line for each of this guidebook's hikes to check conditions prior to heading out for your hike. And don't try to circumvent such closures.

★ Avoid trespassing on private land, and obtain all permits and authorization as required. Also, leave gates as you found them or as directed by signage.

★ Be courteous to other hikers, bikers, equestrians, and others you encounter on the trails.

★ Never spook wild animals or pets. An unannounced approach, a sudden movement, or a loud noise startles most critters, and a surprised animal can be dangerous to you, to others, and to itself. Give animals plenty of space.

★ Observe the YIELD signs around the region's trailheads and back-country. Typically they advise hikers to yield to horses, and bikers to yield to both horses and hikers. Observing common courtesy on hills, hikers and bikers yield to any uphill traffic. When encountering mounted riders or horsepackers, hikers can courteously step off the trail, on the downhill side if possible. So that horses can see and hear you, calmly greet their riders before they reach you, and do not dart behind trees. Also resist the urge to pet horses unless you are invited to do so.

★ Stay on the existing trail and do not blaze any new trails.

★ Be sure to pack out what you pack in, leaving only your footprints. No one likes to see the trash someone else has left behind.

Tips on Enjoying Hiking in Raleigh and Durham

It's easy to enjoy hiking around Raleigh/Durham, but a few tips might enhance the experience. First, check out all of the information listed in this book for the particular trail you consider hiking. Note the contact information and the GPS coordinates of the trailhead. The trail descriptions will help you know what to expect along the trail and help you prepare for such elements as water crossings, fishing opportunities, and views (that is, bring your camera).

The trails around Raleigh/Durham can be fairly spread out since this book covers such a large geographical area. So it's always a good idea to see how far a trail may be from your point of origin to avoid driving an hour to a trail when you really just wanted to do a quick day hike. The terrain around Raleigh/Durham is also very diverse, and you will want to consider your own fitness level when making decisions about what type of physical challenge you want to take on.

Take your time on the trail and don't rush. Hiking presents a great opportunity to relax and think. Hurrying along the trail and becoming too goal oriented with the process can sometimes take away from the experience.

The main point, though, is to get what you want out of the trail. If you want a physical challenge to run the trails, time yourself, and attempt to set new records, do it. If you want to take a whole day to hike a few miles, sitting and picnicking and watching the clouds roll by, then you should set aside a day to do this. Just make sure to hike the trail in your own way and make it *your* experience.

Just as important as it is to never live anyone else's life, you should never hike anyone else's trail.

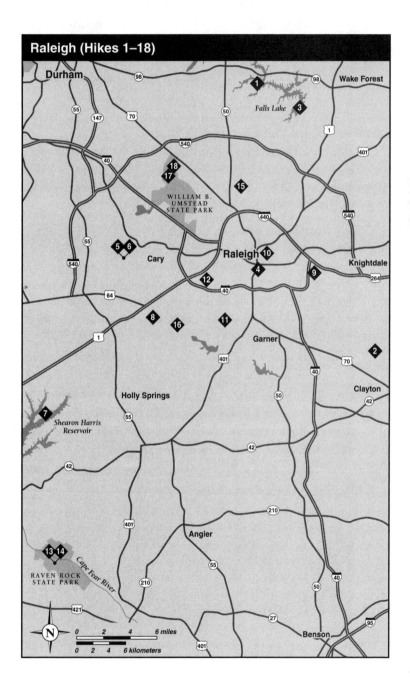

Raleigh (Hikes 1–18)

Raleigh

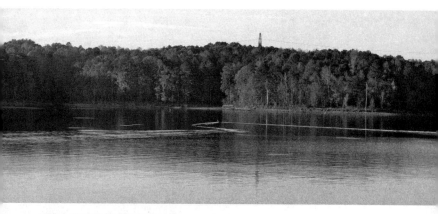

A VIEW OF FALLS LAKE FROM BLUE JAY POINT

Blue Jay Point County Park Loop

SCENERY: ★ ★ ★ ★ ★
TRAIL CONDITION: ★ ★ ★ ★ ★
CHILDREN: ★ ★ ★ ★ ★
DIFFICULTY: ★ ★ ★
SOLITUDE: ★ ★

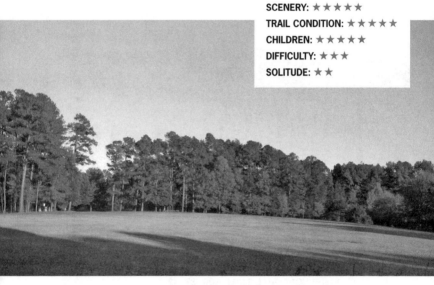

ENJOY THE SPACIOUS RECREATION FIELDS AT BLUE JAY POINT.

GPS TRAILHEAD COORDINATES: N35° 58.173' W78° 38.545'

DISTANCE & CONFIGURATION: 1.6-mile loop

HIKING TIME: 1 hour

HIGHLIGHTS: Blue Jay Point, Falls Lake, playing field, and garden area

ELEVATION: 339' at the trailhead to 246' at lowest point

ACCESS: Trails: Daily, 8 a.m.–sunset. Blue Jay Center for Environmental Education: Daily, 8 a.m.–5 p.m. Closed January 1, Thanksgiving, and December 24–25. Free.

MAPS: Online at wakegov.com/parks

FACILITIES: Restrooms, water fountains, playground, garden, baseball field, and lodge

WHEELCHAIR ACCESS: Not on these trails, but much of the rest of the park is accessible by wheelchair.

COMMENTS: Pets must be kept on a leash no longer than 6 feet. Bikes are not allowed on any of the trails in Blue Jay Point County Park. The park is very popular with school groups and families with children. To avoid crowds, visit on weekday mornings.

CONTACTS: 919-870-4330; wakegov.com/parks

Overview

This loop, combining three popular trails in Blue Jay Point County Park, starts from the visitor center and garden area. From here you cross the park's main road and follow an unpaved footpath through the playing field. You then join the Blue Jay Point Trail on a pleasant walk that traverses small hills and leads to Blue Jay Point, with scenic views of the surrounding Falls Lake. From here the trail backtracks to the Falls Lake Trail and follows along the shore of Falls Lake, passing a short spur trail that leads to Beaver Point, another scenic overlook of the lake. The route then circles back to the northwest on the Beaver Point Trail, which intersects the Azalea Loop Trail before returning to the visitor center and garden area, where you started.

Route Details

Blue Jay Point County Park is a 236-acre park bordered on three sides by Falls Lake, Raleigh's primary drinking-water supply. The area was once mostly agricultural land, but now you find second-growth forests. Nestled in this forest, 3 acres of the park are dedicated to open playing fields, playgrounds, an environmental-education center, and an overnight lodge. Five miles of trails crisscross the park, the longest being the 3.1-mile Falls Lake Trail.

The park officially opened o the public on January 1, 1992, and is focused on environmental education. The Blue Jay Center for Environmental Education is an exhibit hall and classroom center that explores environmental topics. A lodge near Sandy Point in the northern part of the park can be reserved by organizations for overnight environmental-education programs.

Park your vehicle in the visitor-center parking lot. In front of the building and across the paved road is a wooden staircase. Walk up the staircase and follow the 2-foot-wide unpaved path through the beautiful playing field. This is a perfect spot to enjoy a picnic or to throw the Frisbee around; a playground is to the left. To the southeast, in the right back corner of the field, walk down the staircase that leads

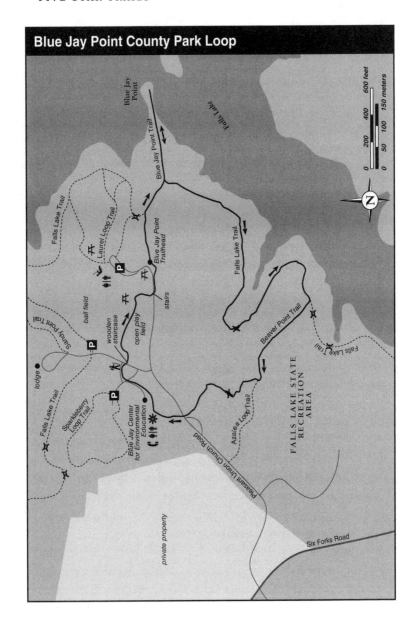

Blue Jay Point County Park Loop

to the paved road. Cross the paved road and turn left (east) toward the traffic circle and continue to the Blue Jay Point Trailhead.

Follow the gravel trail, blazed with blue dots, into the forest. The trail leads downhill for 0.3 mile, passing the junction with the Falls Lake Trail and continuing downhill to Blue Jay Point, with incredible scenic views of the lake that surrounds the peninsula. After exploring and enjoying the point, turn around and backtrack to the junction with the Falls Lake Trail, 0.1 mile away. Turn left (south) onto the Falls Lake Trail, blazed with white circles, and follow the 3-foot-wide unpaved path through the forest and along the shore of the lake, keeping the lake to your left.

Continue 0.3 mile and cross the wooden footbridge over the creek. From here the trail climbs uphill, and after 0.2 mile you reach the intersection with the Beaver Point Trail, a short spur leading to Beaver Point and more great views of Falls Lake. Turn right (northwest) and follow the unpaved, 10-foot-wide Beaver Point Trail uphill for 0.1 mile until you reach the junction with the 0.4-mile-long Azalea Loop Trail. Turn right (northeast) and follow the Azalea Loop Trail for 250 feet, descending the 4-foot-wide unpaved path to a creek. Cross the wooden footbridge over the creek and then

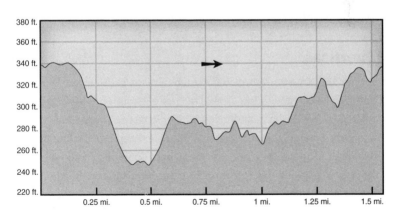

hike up the hill to the paved road, 450 feet away. Cross the paved road, Pleasant Union Church Road, and pass through the garden area, following the gravel road for 0.1 mile that leads back to the visitor center and the parking lot where you started.

Nearby Attractions

Falls Lake State Recreation Area, with a 12,000-acre lake and 26,000 acres of woodlands, offers more than 20 miles of hiking trails, including a portion of the Mountains-to-Sea Trail traversing the south shore of the lake, as well as other shorter trails at Beaver Dam, B. W. Wells, Holly Point, Rolling View, and Sandling Beach. The 1-mile loop trail at B. W. Wells passes the naturalist's home (see page 163). The entrance to Falls Lake State Recreation Area is 4 miles northwest of the Blue Jay Point County Park.

At the southeast end of the lake, 6 miles southeast of the Blue Jay Point County Park, is the Falls Lake Visitor Assistance Center (see page 39). A 1-mile unpaved nature trail connects with the longer Falls Lake Trail that runs for 38 miles, from the Tailrace Fishing Area below Falls Dam, along the southern shore of the lake, and to the Rolling View State Recreation Area. The park also has a 2-mile paved walking trail that borders the entrance road.

Directions

From Raleigh, go northeast on Capital Boulevard/US 70 toward West Johnson Street, and follow Capital 8.3 miles. Merge onto I-540 West toward US 70/Durham, and follow the interstate 5.2 miles. Take the Six Forks Road exit, Exit 11, and go 0.2 mile. Keep right, taking the Six Forks Road north ramp, and merge onto Six Forks Road. Follow Six Forks Road 2.4 miles. Turn left to stay on Six Forks Road, and follow it an additional 1.5 miles. Turn right onto Pleasant Union Church Road, and follow it 0.3 mile until you reach the entrance to Blue Jay Point County Park.

From Durham, start out going east on Holloway Street/NC 98 toward North Queen Street. Continue to follow NC 98 for 13.7 miles. Turn right onto Six Forks Road and follow it 1.5 miles. Turn left onto Pleasant Union Church Road and follow it 0.3 mile until you reach the entrance to Blue Jay Point County Park.

Clemmons Educational State Forest

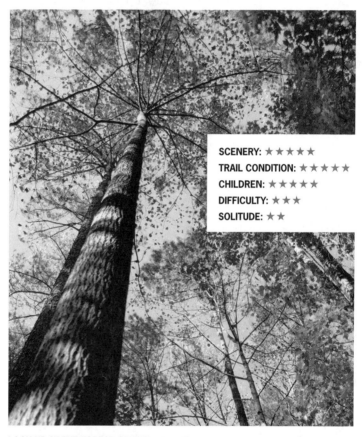

SCENERY: ★ ★ ★ ★ ★
TRAIL CONDITION: ★ ★ ★ ★ ★
CHILDREN: ★ ★ ★ ★ ★
DIFFICULTY: ★ ★
SOLITUDE: ★ ★

LOOK UP AT THE FOREST CANOPY AT CLEMMONS EDUCATIONAL STATE FOREST.

GPS TRAILHEAD COORDINATES: N35° 58.173' W78° 38.545'

DISTANCE & CONFIGURATION: 2.7-mile loop

HIKING TIME: 2 hours

HIGHLIGHTS: Interpretive displays, pine stands, rock formations, and creeks

ELEVATION: 260' at trailhead to 300' at peak and 173' at lowest point

ACCESS: Mid-March–mid-November: Tuesday–Friday, 9 a.m.–5 p.m.; Saturday–Sunday, 11 a.m.–5 p.m.

MAPS: Online at ncesf.org, at the on-site visitor center, and at the trailhead kiosk

FACILITIES: Restrooms, water fountains, educational center, and picnic pavilions

WHEELCHAIR ACCESS: Sections of the trail near the parking lot and the path to the picnic shelter are paved and accessible to wheelchairs. However, most of the trail system is unpaved and inaccessible.

COMMENTS: The trail is very popular with children and large school groups, so if you're in need of solitude, you may want to look elsewhere. The park has strict policies for dog— they must be leashed at all times, and the owner must be in full control of the pet. Bikes and motorized vehicles are *not* allowed on any of the trails in the forest.

CONTACTS: 919-553-5651; ncesf.org

Overview

Clemmons Educational State Forest lies 16 miles southeast of Raleigh, between the Piedmont and the coastal plain. The Clemmons's pine stands and hardwoods are set on a rolling terrain that is highlighted by streams and rock formations. This was the first designated North Carolina educational state forest, and throughout it you encounter interactive interpretive stations that describe the forest's ecology, geology, history, and management techniques through fun anecdotal recordings and displays. While the displays are geared toward children, they are still very enjoyable and interesting for adults.

This route combines three of the four trails in the forest— the Talking Tree Trail, the Talking Rock Trail, and the Demonstration Trail—to make a loop that explores a significant portion of the park. The trail starts near a spacious picnic pavilion with tables surrounding a wide stone fireplace, where you are likely to find a fire burning during the cooler months. From here the Talking Tree Trail winds its way through a forest of gentle rolling hills and crosses streams, while along the way you learn about the natural history of the trees in the forest through prerecorded messages at the interpretive stations.

This route circles back around to briefly follow the Talking Rock Trail and encounter a few fine examples of stone specimens at the interpretive stations. The path then makes a 1.9-mile loop, following the Demonstration Trail over larger hills and through a managed

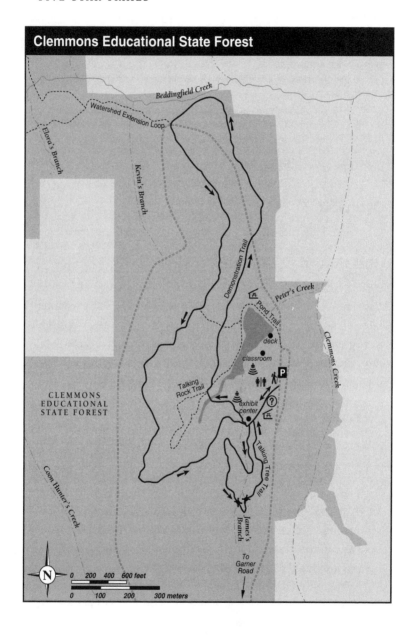

Clemmons Educational State Forest

pine forest, with interpretive stations that describe and illustrate the techniques used in forest management and harvesting.

Route Details

Follow the gravel road to the parking lot at the north end of the park. The trailhead is on the west side of the parking lot, next to the lookout tower. Follow the 8-foot-wide paved trail past the cross-section display of the 220-year-old southern red oak. It is quite impressive and allows you to visualize what the old-growth forest must have looked like in the 1700s before it was harvested. After 0.1 mile you reach an interpretive kiosk on your left (south), where the trail splits four ways.

Turn right (west) and continue on the paved path, which quickly turns unpaved and leads to the main kiosk and Talking Tree Trailhead. At the kiosk, turn left (south), and after 60 feet the trail splits. Stay to the left (south) on the Talking Tree Trail, heading toward the octagonal, wooden-sided exhibit center. Continue for 350 feet until you reach a split in the trail. Stay to the left (southwest) and continue on the green-diamond-blazed Talking Tree Trail.

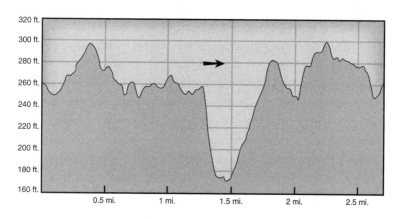

You start to encounter the interpretive stations—colorfully painted speaker boxes—along this section of the trail. Simply push the red button, and you will hear a recording that describes the natural history of the trees in the forest. A forest-service symbol indicates the tree described by each interpretive station, so you can relate the recorded message to the actual tree featured. The recorded messages are very well produced and are especially interesting for young children.

The trail crosses a creek over a small wooden footbridge and then veers to the right. Continue through the forest and cross the larger wooden bridge. Interpretive stations along the way describe a variety of trees in detail, including loblolly pine, white cedar, sugar gum, and red cedar trees. After 0.2 mile you reach a gravel trail. Turn left (west) and continue again toward the exhibit center and the trailhead to the 2.2-mile Demonstration Trail. Once you reach the well-marked trailhead, keep to the left on the red-diamond-blazed Demonstration Trail. After just 15 feet the trail splits. Stay to the right (west). After just another 130 feet, the trail splits again. Stay to the right (northwest) on the 3-foot-wide unpaved trail.

You can find clues that will reveal the history of this forest if you know where to look. At the base of the stumps of some of the longleaf pine trees, you will see scars that were left in the Colonial period, when the sap from these trees was harvested and used to seal the hulls of wooden boats and ships. The sap was also collected and turned into turpentine, resin, pitch, and tar. Furrows can be seen here and there throughout the forest as well—these are testament to the farming that was practiced in the 20th century, when these forests were fields. Before this land was designated as an educational forest in 1976, it was used as a nursery, constructed by the Civilian Conservation Corps in the 1930s and later run by the North Carolina Division of Forest Resources.

During this next section the Demonstration Trail merges with the Talking Rock Trail, and you get the opportunity to explore some of the geology-focused interpretive stations. The trail passes a large example of limestone and then descends to a wooden walkway that crosses a rocky and cascading stream. When you reach the trail junction, the Talking Rock Trail continues to the left. However, stay to the right (north) and continue on the Demonstration Trail. After almost 100 feet you reach a trail junction. To the right the Pond Trail descends to the pond. However, stay to the left (north) and ascend the hill, staying on the red-blazed Demonstration Trail.

After 0.1 mile you reach a four-way intersection. If you want to make this hike 0.7 mile shorter, you can turn left (west) and take this shortcut trail to the other side of the Demonstration Trail loop. To continue on the entire loop, stay straight (north). Over this next section of trail you cross some larger rolling hills, but they are still only moderately challenging. Continue for 0.2 mile until you cross the dirt road. The trail begins to gradually descend to a beautiful area of the forest, where you will see an abundance of ferns in the understory. Here the trail turns to the left (west) and runs beside the shallow, sandy-bottomed creek.

The trail bends to the left (south) and crosses the dirt road again. Continue on the Demonstration Trail for 1 mile until you reach the octagonal exhibit center again. Turn right (southeast) and follow the trail around the exhibit center, then continue following the gravel trail back to the parking lot, the trailhead, and the end of the hike.

Nearby Attractions

The 0.5-mile Pond Trail is the only other trail in Clemmons Educational State Forest, but 9 miles to the north is Historic Oak View County Park (see page 71), a 19th-century historic farmstead that you can explore along brick paved paths. The park has artfully preserved farmhouses, gardens, barns, and even a few friendly goats to visit. It's free and well worth the trip.

Historic Yates Mill County Park (see page 82) is 14 miles west of Clemmons Educational State Forest. You can explore more than 2 miles of trails that follow along the creek and circle a large pond in the center of the park. Visit the historic Yates Mill, opened in 1750 and the only remaining Wake County gristmill in working condition.

Directions

From Raleigh, take I-40 East and follow it 7 miles. Merge onto US 70 East via Exit 306 toward Clayton, and follow it 4 miles. Turn sharply to the left onto Guy Road and follow it 0.4 mile. Turn right onto East Garner Road and follow it 1.1 miles. After East Garner Road becomes Old US 70 West, continue another 0.9 mile until you reach the entrance to Clemmons Educational State Forest. If you reach Powell Drive, you've gone about 0.4 mile too far.

Falls Lake Visitor Assistance Center:
Falls Lake Trail

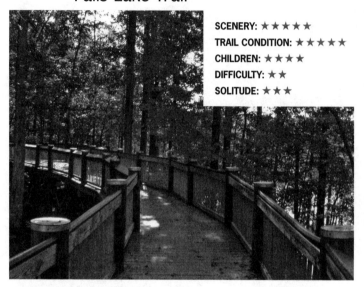

SCENERY: ★ ★ ★ ★
TRAIL CONDITION: ★ ★ ★ ★ ★
CHILDREN: ★ ★ ★ ★
DIFFICULTY: ★ ★
SOLITUDE: ★ ★ ★

A BOARDWALK LINES THE LAKESHORE AT THE FALLS LAKE VISITOR ASSISTANCE CENTER.

GPS TRAILHEAD COORDINATES: N35° 56.327' W78° 35.189'

DISTANCE & CONFIGURATION: 0.9-mile loop

HIKING TIME: 1 hour

HIGHLIGHTS: Falls Lake, Falls Lake Visitor Assistance Center, and hardwood-and-pine forest

ELEVATION: 278' at trailhead to 337' at peak

ACCESS: October–March: Monday–Friday, 8 a.m.–4:30 p.m. April–September: Daily, 8 a.m.–4:30 p.m. Free.

MAPS: Online at www.saw.usace.army.mil/falls/TrailMapV3Website.pdf and at the Visitor Assistance Center

FACILITIES: Restrooms, environmental-education center, picnic area, and water fountains

WHEELCHAIR ACCESS: None

COMMENTS: Dogs are allowed in the park as long as they are kept on a leash of 6 feet or less. The trails are popular with runners, especially the paved trails that follow the park entrance road.

CONTACTS: 919-846-9332, ext. 224; eenorthcarolina.org; www.saw.usace.army.mil/falls

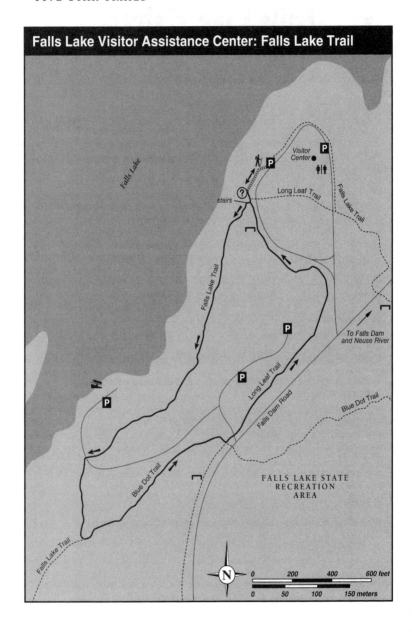

Falls Lake Visitor Assistance Center: Falls Lake Trail

Falls Lake

Visitor Center

Long Leaf Trail

stairs

Falls Lake Trail

Falls Lake Trail

To Falls Dam
and Neuse River

Long Leaf Trail

Falls Dam Road

Blue Dot Trail

Blue Dot Trail

FALLS LAKE STATE
RECREATION
AREA

Falls Lake Trail

N

| 0 | 200 | 400 | 600 feet |

| 0 | 50 | 100 | 150 meters |

Overview

This trail follows along the southeast shore of Falls Lake and explores the hardwood forest and pine stands that surround the lake. The trail starts at the Falls Lake Visitor Assistance Center, which contains the dam and emergency spillway. From here the trail follows the shore of the lake along an elevated boardwalk that offers views of the surrounding water. The route then follows an unpaved path through a pine-and-hardwood forest along the lake. The path loops around to join a paved walking trail and returns to the Falls Lake Visitor Assistance Center, which offers exhibits on fish and wildlife conservation, water quality, and the construction and operation of the dam.

Route Details

Falls Lake is a 12,000-acre artificial reservoir on the upper portion of North Carolina's Neuse River Basin, which extends 22 miles upstream from the dam to the convergence of the Eno and Flat Rivers near Durham. The Falls project was authorized for flood control, water supply, water quality, and recreation. At its deepest point, at Falls Dam, the lake is 51.5 feet deep. However, most of the lake is comparatively shallow, averaging only 10–20 feet deep, and the upper end of the lake averages only 5–6 feet deep.

Around the lake you will find a variety of recreation opportunities apart from the hiking trails, including swimming beaches, campgrounds, picnic pavilions, boat ramps, and fishing piers. Surrounding the lake are 26,000 acres of public land that provide vital habitat for several rare and endangered species, including the bald eagle and the smooth coneflower. The falls that are referred to in the park's name were actually covered up when the US Army Corps of Engineers flooded the surrounding valley to make the Falls Lake Reservoir. There are still some smaller falls south of the Falls Lake Reservoir Dam, but the falls that gave the nearby neighborhood of Lake Falls its name are now underneath the surface of the lake.

Along this trail you will briefly join the Falls Lake Trail, which currently runs for 38 miles from the Tailrace Fishing Area below Falls Lake Reservoir Dam, along the southern shore of the lake, and to the Rolling View Recreation Area. The trail is part of the North Carolina Mountains-to-Sea Trail and will eventually run for approximately 60 miles all the way up to the Eno River, and past I-85.

Drive to the Falls Lake Visitor Assistance Center and park your vehicle in the lot near the center. You can pick up a map of the park inside the center. The trailhead is behind the visitor center, on the west side of the parking lot. Walk on the nicely constructed elevated boardwalk for 215 feet until you reach the kiosk. An unpaved path heads straight (south). However, turn right and follow the wooden steps down to the 3-foot-wide unpaved path that follows along the shore of the lake. Falls Lake Trail is blazed with white circles and continues through a beautiful mature forest. Continue for 0.3 mile until you reach the paved road. Turn left (east) onto the Blue Dot Trail.

Continue straight (east) for 500 feet, following the Blue Dot Trail as it curves around to the right (south), until you reach the park's paved entrance road. Turn left (northeast) onto the paved path, called the Long Leaf Trail, which follows alongside the entrance road. Follow the Long Leaf Trail the entire way back to the Falls Lake Visitor Assistance Center, the parking lot where you started, and the end of the hike.

Nearby Attractions

Falls Lake State Recreation Area, with a 12,000-acre lake and 26,000 acres of woodlands, offers more than 20 miles of hiking trails along the portion of the Mountains-to-Sea Trail that traverses the south shore of the lake, as well as along other shorter trails at Beaverdam, B. W. Wells, Holly Point, Rolling View, and Sandling Beach. The 1-mile loop at B. W. Wells passes the naturalist's home (see page 163). The entrance to Falls Lake State Recreation Area is 12 miles northwest of the Falls Lake Visitor Assistance Center.

Blue Jay Point County Park, a 236-acre park on the shores of Falls Lake in northern Wake County, offers more than 5 miles of trails within its boundaries, as well as open play fields, playgrounds, an environmental education center, and an overnight lodge. The park (see page 26) features hiking trails that also connect with the Falls Lake State Recreation Area trails to offer longer hiking opportunities. The park is 6 miles northwest of the Falls Lake Visitor Assistance Center.

Directions

From Raleigh, start out going northeast on Capital Boulevard/US 70 toward West Johnson Street and follow it 8.3 miles. Merge onto I-540 West toward US 70/Durham and follow it 2.9 miles. Take the Falls of Neuse Road exit, Exit 14, and follow the road 0.2 mile. Turn left onto Falls of Neuse Road and follow it 2.5 miles. Turn left onto Falls Dam Road and follow the signs to the Falls Lake Visitor Assistance Center. Park in the lot in front of the visitor center, and follow the sidewalk to the trailhead at the start of the boardwalk.

From Durham, take Holloway Street/US 70 Bypass Road East and follow it 19.7 miles. Turn right onto Falls of Neuse Road and follow it 3.6 miles. Turn right onto Falls Dam Road and follow the signs to the Falls Lake Visitor Assistance Center. Park in the lot in front of the visitor center, and follow the sidewalk to the trailhead, at the start of the boardwalk.

Fayetteville Street and City Market Walk

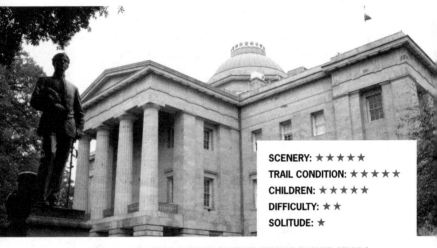

SCENERY: ★ ★ ★ ★ ★
TRAIL CONDITION: ★ ★ ★ ★ ★
CHILDREN: ★ ★ ★ ★ ★
DIFFICULTY: ★ ★
SOLITUDE: ★

THE *WORTH BAGLEY MONUMENT* BY FRANCIS HERMAN PACKER STANDS
BEFORE THE NORTH CAROLINA STATE CAPITOL.

GPS TRAILHEAD COORDINATES: N35° 46.382' W78° 38.372'

DISTANCE & CONFIGURATION: 1.8-mile loop

HIKING TIME: 1.5 hours

HIGHLIGHTS: City Market, Fayetteville Street, State Capitol, and the North Carolina
Museum of Natural Sciences

ELEVATION: 334' at trailhead to 356' at peak and 305' at lowest point

ACCESS: 24/7, but not recommended late at night; free

MAPS: Online at visitraleigh.com or at the Raleigh Visitor Information Center, in the
Raleigh Marriott City Center hotel

FACILITIES: Restrooms and water fountains

WHEELCHAIR ACCESS: Yes

COMMENTS: The Raleigh Visitor Information Center is inside the Fayetteville Street
Downtown Marriott Hotel at Fayetteville Street. The center can be a little difficult to find.
There are no signs directing you to it once you go inside the hotel. Simply enter the hotel,
turn left, and then take your first right. Follow the steps down to the visitor center, which is
straight ahead through the double doors. Dogs are allowed in downtown Raleigh as long as
they are kept on a leash no longer than 6 feet.

CONTACTS: 919-833-1120; visitraleigh.com

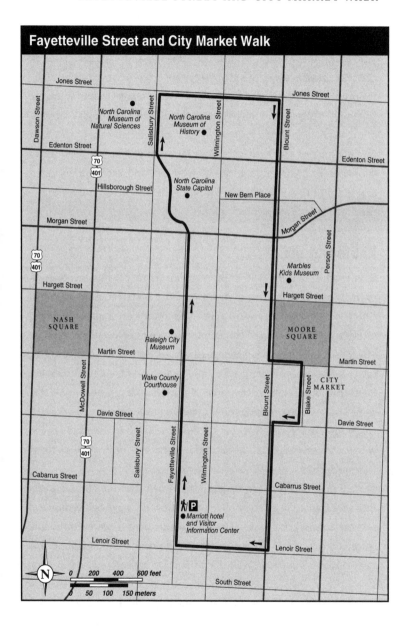

Fayetteville Street and City Market Walk

Overview

This walk takes you into downtown Raleigh and explores some of the best attractions in the area. The walk starts at the Raleigh Visitor Information Center, at the Raleigh Marriott City Center hotel on Fayetteville Street, and walks up Fayetteville Street through the heart of the business district. From here the trail leads past the State Capitol building and the North Carolina Museum of Natural Sciences. A short detour leads through the City Market and explores the cafés and shops of the pedestrian-only area of the city before you return to the Marriott at Raleigh's city center.

Route Details

Stop by the Raleigh Visitor Information Center and grab a map of downtown. The route starts in front of the Marriott. Standing outside the Marriott on Fayetteville Street, turn left (north) on Fayetteville and walk toward the Capitol, four blocks away. Fayetteville Street is considered the central business district of Raleigh, and the towering skyscrapers define Raleigh as a distinctive and successful Southern city, while the restored historic buildings that share the same space along this main downtown road keep the city reverently charming. Fayetteville Street is also known as Raleigh's Grand Boulevard, adorned with public art, outdoor cafés, and impressive 28-foot-wide sidewalks.

Raleigh really began downtown. Named after the 16th-century English explorer Sir Walter Raleigh, downtown Raleigh had commerce as early as the 1760s. Isaac Hunter and Joel Lane, two enterprising landholders, created taverns and founded primitive inns around the early outpost known as Wake Crossroads to accommodate travelers along the main north–south route cutting through central North Carolina. This was the spark that eventually would ignite commerce in the region, and it would grow into what you see today along Fayetteville Street.

After walking two blocks, you'll pass the Wake County Courthouse on the left. Continue on Fayetteville Street until the road abruptly dead-ends and leaves you facing the stunning cross-shaped building featuring a central, domed rotunda—this is the North Carolina State Capitol. A National Historic Landmark, the Capitol building was completed in 1840 and is constructed in the Greek Revival style of architecture. Guided tours of the Capitol are available on Saturday, 11 a.m.–2 p.m. On weekdays you are welcome to take a free self-guided tour.

Follow the paved path around to the left of the Capitol until you reach Jones Street. Turn right (east) onto Jones Street and pass the North Carolina Museum of Natural Sciences and the North Carolina Museum of History. Admission is free to both of these museums, and they are highly recommended. The Capital Area Visitor Center, an information and rest center, is in the lobby of the North Carolina Museum of History.

Walk 0.2 mile, crossing Wilmington Street, and turn right (south) onto Blount Street. Continue for 0.4 mile, or four blocks, along Blount Street, passing the Marbles Kids Museum and Imax theater on the left between Morgan and Hargett Streets. Admission to the Marbles Kids Museum is $5, and the museum has all types of hands-on exhibits where children can learn and play at the same time.

Turn left (west) onto Martin Street and continue for 160 feet. Cross Martin, via the crosswalk, to enter into the City Market, opened in 1914. Today the charm of the historic shopping district is still captured in the classic brick buildings that line the cobblestone streets. Recommended stops are the gallery at Artspace, Big Ed's restaurant, Vic's Italian Restaurant & Pizzeria, Woody's, Benelux Café, and Rum Runners. If you're here on the first Friday of each month, the stores stay open for extended hours, and crowds come out to tour the art galleries and listen to live bands that perform in front of the shops in the market. It's a fun community event, and there is often free wine.

After passing through the City Market, turn right (west) onto Davie Street toward Blount Street. Here you enter into the district that is known as East Raleigh, or South Park. Once you reach Blount Street, turn left (south), continue for two blocks, or 0.2 mile, and turn left (west) on Lenoir Street. From here you just have to walk two blocks, cross Fayetteville Street, and return to the Marriott where you started.

Nearby Attractions

The historic Oakwood neighborhood is only 0.5 mile north of the downtown Marriott at Raleigh's city center. The Oakwood neighborhood (see page 76) is listed on the National Register of Historic Places and has the finest examples of 19th-century homes in the region. The governor's executive mansion is at the southwestern border of the historic neighborhood, and the area also features the historic Oakwood Inn Bed & Breakfast, Oakwood Cemetery, and houses developed by Colonel Jonathan Heck.

The Mordecai Historic Park (919-857-4364), at 1 Mimosa St., is just 1.5 miles north of the Marriott and makes a great addition to a day of touring downtown Raleigh. Inside the park are the best-preserved homes in Raleigh's most historic neighborhood. Admission to the park, which includes a 1-hour tour, is just $5 for adults and $3 for children and seniors. Tours are offered Tuesday–Sunday, but the park grounds are open daily, sunrise–sunset.

Directions

From the Fayetteville area, take I-95 North and follow it 26.1 miles. Merge onto I-40 West via Exit 81 toward Raleigh and follow it 29.5 miles. Take the Hammond Road exit, Exit 299, toward Person Street. Keep right to take the ramp toward Person Street/Shaw University. Merge onto Hammond Road and follow it 1.1 miles. Turn left onto East Lenoir Street and follow it 0.2 mile. Turn right onto Fayetteville Street and follow it 0.1 mile. The Marriott hotel and visitor center, at 500 Fayetteville St., is on the left; if you reach Hanover Square, you've gone too far.

From the Durham area, take I-40 East toward Raleigh-Durham International Airport and follow it 9.6 miles. Merge onto Wade Avenue via Exit 289 toward I-440/US 1 North and follow it 2.1 miles. Take the Blue Ridge Road exit and follow it 0.3 mile. Turn right onto Blue Ridge Road and follow it 1.3 miles. Turn left onto Western Boulevard and follow it 3.6 miles. Merge onto South McDowell Street and follow it 0.5 mile. Turn right onto West Lenoir Street and follow it 0.1 mile. Turn left onto Fayetteville Street and follow it 0.1 mile. The Marriott and visitor center, at 500 Fayetteville St., is on the left; if you reach Hanover Square, you've gone too far.

5

Fred G. Bond
Metro Park: Lake Trail

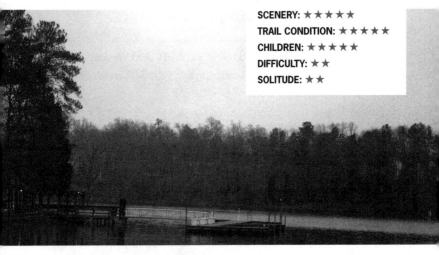

SCENERY: ★ ★ ★ ★ ★
TRAIL CONDITION: ★ ★ ★ ★ ★
CHILDREN: ★ ★ ★ ★ ★
DIFFICULTY: ★ ★
SOLITUDE: ★ ★

BOND LAKE ON A FOGGY MORNING

GPS TRAILHEAD COORDINATES: N35° 46.920' W78° 49.407'

DISTANCE & CONFIGURATION: 2.1-mile loop

HIKING TIME: 1.5 hours

HIGHLIGHTS: Bond Lake and activity field

ELEVATION: 385' at trailhead to 331' at lowest point

ACCESS: November–February: Daily, 9 a.m.–6 p.m. March: Daily, 9 a.m.–7 p.m. April–May and September–October: Sunday–Friday, 9 a.m.–8 p.m.; Saturday and holidays, 8 a.m.–8 p.m. June–August: Sunday–Friday, 9 a.m.–9 p.m.; Saturday and holidays, 7 a.m.–9 p.m. Free.

MAPS: Online at townofcary.org, at trailhead kiosks, or at the park's boathouse and community center

FACILITIES: Restrooms, water fountains, playground, sports fields, ropes course, community center, senior center, picnic pavilions, and boat rentals

WHEELCHAIR ACCESS: None on this trail, although other areas of the park and some of the other trails are.

COMMENTS: This is a very popular park in Cary, and the paved sections of the trails are very popular with bikers. To avoid collisions, be alert for other runners and bikers when walking these trails. Leashed dogs are allowed in the park.

CONTACTS: 919-469-4100; townofcary.org

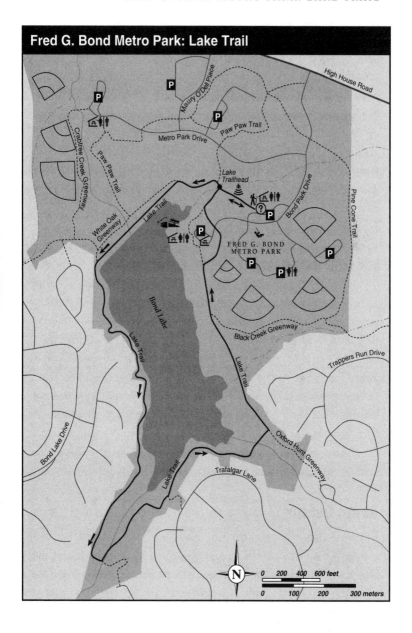

Fred G. Bond Metro Park: Lake Trail

Overview

Fred G. Bond Metro Park is in east Cary, 12 miles west of Raleigh. It's about a 20-minute drive from Raleigh to the park. Fred G. Bond Metro Park is the one-stop shop for outdoor recreation in Cary. The 310-acre park has more than 4 miles of hiking trails that are focused around Bond Lake. All of the trails in the park share a centralized trailhead near the north end of Bond Lake. The Black Creek Greenway, Oxford Hunt Greenway, and White Oak Greenway all intersect at Fred G. Bond Metro Park. The park has eight sports fields, a large general activity field, a senior center, a community center with basketball courts, and an outdoor amphitheater. You can even rent a boat to take out on the lake from the boathouse located on the northeast side of Bond Lake.

The Lake Trail circumnavigates the entire shoreline of Bond Lake. It is an easy trail and great for runners. The views of the lake can at times be stunning, and the trail is well maintained and easy to follow. It is a great trail for children who are up for a 2-mile hike. The trail starts from the north end of the lake and follows along a gravel-top berm on the northwest side of the lake before entering into a dense forest. The trail often passes behind houses that line the lakeshore on the south end of the lake, and several spur trails lead from the lakeshore into the nearby neighborhood. The trail crosses a short dam on the south end of the lake before passing by an exercise station and a playground and returning to the trailhead.

Route Details

Follow the park signs to the Kiwanis shelter and park at the shelter lot. A map kiosk at the west corner of the parking lot marks the beginning of the spur trail that leads to the centralized trailhead for all of the trails in the park. Near the kiosk are restrooms and a large picnic pavilion at the north end of the parking lot. Follow the dirt path to the left (west) of the kiosk and down the short hill to the large amphitheater. The paved trail behind the amphitheater leads to the large, blue-roofed kiosk that serves as the centralized trailhead for the park.

From the trailhead turn left (southwest) and follow the Lake Trail toward the lake. You pass a large general activity field on the right. This is a great spot to picnic, fly a kite, or throw a Frisbee or football around, and most days you'll see plenty of people enjoying this great space. Continue following the paved path for 400 feet until you reach a junction in the trail. Veer left (south), leaving the paved path and following the gravel trail up onto the narrow berm that follows along the lake's northwestern shore. All along the berm you have excellent views of the lake, and if you are looking for an exceptionally short trail, the end of the berm is a great place to turn around.

To complete the entire 2-mile loop, follow along the top of the berm for 0.2 mile until you reach a split in the trail. Stay straight (south) and continue following the dirt path along the lakeshore. Continue on the 4-foot-wide dirt path that follows along the lakeshore for 0.7 mile. Along this section, the trail follows behind several homes before leaving the lake behind and entering into a dense pine-and-oak forest. The trail curves around to the east at the south end of Bond Lake before reaching a trail junction. Stay straight (northeast) and follow the trail through the forest and back toward the lake. Continue walking through the forest for 0.4 mile until you reach another trail junction. Turn left (northeast) onto the paved path and continue toward the lake.

The 7-foot-wide paved path rejoins the lakeshore and continues for 0.5 mile, passing a set of monkey bars on the right. When you reach the boathouse parking lot, veer right and cross the road. Continue on the paved path to the amphitheater on the right, and finally reach the centralized trailhead, kiosk, and the end of the trail.

Nearby Attractions

Hemlock Bluffs Nature Preserve (see page 66) is 4 miles to the west of Fred G. Bond Metro Park and has almost 4 miles of hiking trails. The trails in Hemlock Bluffs are slightly more challenging than the trails at Bond Park. The trails at Hemlock traverse small hills and lead to steep bluffs with views of Swift Creek below. The park is designated to protect clusters of eastern hemlocks on the north-facing bluffs and features a nature center geared toward young children.

Swift Creek Bluffs Nature Preserve (see page 111) is in southeast Cary, 6 miles southeast of Fred G. Bond Metro Park. The 23-acre preserve has a 1.2-mile trail that follows along Swift Creek to the bluffs.

Directions

From Raleigh follow Capital Boulevard/US 70 East for 2.2 miles and merge onto I-40 West toward Cary. Follow I-40 West for 7.2 miles. Take NC 54, Exit 290, toward Cary and follow NC 54 for 0.2 mile. Turn left onto Chapel Hill Road/NC 54 West and follow it 1.2 miles. Turn right onto northeast Maynard Road/NC 54 West and follow it 3.7 miles. Turn right onto High House Road and follow it 0.7 mile until you reach 801 High House Road and the entrance to Fred G. Bond Metro Park, on the left.

6

Fred G. Bond Metro Park:
Paw Paw and Pine Cone Trails

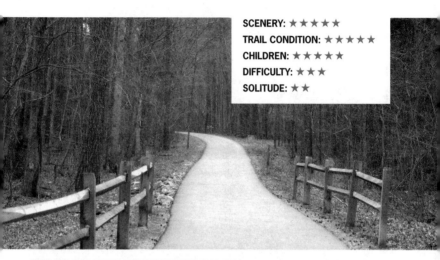

SCENERY: ★ ★ ★ ★ ★
TRAIL CONDITION: ★ ★ ★ ★ ★
CHILDREN: ★ ★ ★ ★ ★
DIFFICULTY: ★ ★ ★
SOLITUDE: ★ ★

EXPLORE THE ABUNDANT RECREATION FACILITIES AND THE SURROUNDING FOREST ALONG THE PAW PAW AND PINE CONE TRAILS.

GPS TRAILHEAD COORDINATES: N35° 46.920' W78° 49.410'

DISTANCE & CONFIGURATION: 1.9-mile loop

HIKING TIME: 1.5 hours

HIGHLIGHTS: Bond Lake, sports fields, and pine and oak forest

ELEVATION: 423' at trailhead to 518' at peak and 268' at lowest point

ACCESS: November–February: Daily, 9 a.m.–6 p.m. March: Daily, 9 a.m.–7 p.m. April–May and September–October: Sunday–Friday, 9 a.m.–8 p.m.; Saturday and holidays, 8 a.m.–8 p.m. June–August: Sunday–Friday, 9 a.m.–9 p.m.; Saturday and holidays, 7 a.m.–9 p.m. Free.

MAPS: Online at townofcary.org, at trailhead kiosks, and at the park's boathouse and community center

FACILITIES: Restrooms, water fountains, playground, sports fields, ropes course, community center, senior center, picnic pavilions, and boat rentals

WHEELCHAIR ACCESS: The Paw Paw and Pine Cone Trails are not wheelchair-accessible, although other areas of the park and some of the other trails are.

COMMENTS: This is a very popular park in Cary, and the paved sections of the trails are very popular with bikers. To avoid collisions, be alert for other runners and bikers when walking these trails. Leashed dogs are allowed in the park.

CONTACTS: 919-469-4100; townofcary.org

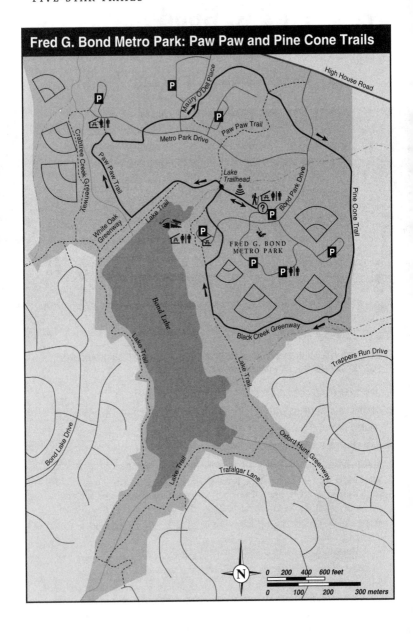

Fred G. Bond Metro Park: Paw Paw and Pine Cone Trails

Overview

This hike combines two trails in Fred G. Bond Metro Park, the Paw Paw Trail and the Pine Cone Trail, to form a 1.9-mile loop. The trail starts in the Kiwanis shelter parking lot and follows along the shore of Bond Lake before entering into a pine-and-oak forest that surrounds the lake. Along the trail you pass the community center with restrooms, basketball courts, and a fitness center. You also will pass by four of the seven sports fields in the park. This loop trail is slightly more challenging than the Lake Trail. It traverses some small hills that are mostly concentrated toward the end of the hike. This enjoyable hike exposes you to most of the park.

Route Details

Follow the park signs to the Kiwanis shelter and park at the shelter lot. A map kiosk at the west corner of the parking lot marks the beginning of the spur trail that leads to a centralized trailhead for all of the trails in the park. Near the kiosk there are restrooms and a large picnic pavilion at the north end of the parking lot. Follow the dirt path to the left

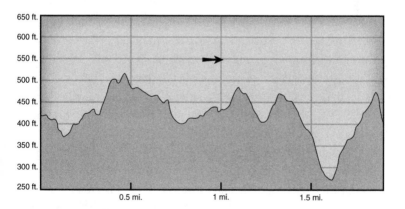

(west) of the kiosk and down the short hill to the large amphitheater. The paved trail behind the amphitheater leads to the large, blue-roofed kiosk that serves as the centralized trailhead of the park.

From the trailhead turn left (southwest) and follow the Lake Trail toward the lake. You pass a large general activity field on the right. This is a great spot to picnic, fly a kite, or throw a Frisbee or football around. Continue following the paved path for 400 feet until you reach a junction in the trail. The lake is to your left, and the Lake Trail follows the gravel trail up onto the berm on the lakeshore. However, for this hike you stay on the paved Paw Paw Trail until you reach the trail junction where the Paw Paw Trail turns to the right and heads away from the lake and into the forest. Turn right (northwest) onto the 4-foot-wide dirt path.

The trail continues to curve around to the right (east) and reaches an intersection. Stay straight (northeast) and continue on the Paw Paw. Over the next 0.2 mile the Paw Paw Trail crosses two paved roads, first Metro Park Drive and then Maury O'Dell Place, and passes behind the community center before reaching another trail junction. Turn left (northeast) and continue on the 4-foot-wide Paw Paw Trail and continue for 0.2 mile until you reach a four-way intersection. If you turn right, you continue on the Paw Paw Trail and back to the main trailhead. If you want or need to make this hike shorter, this is a good way to get back to the trailhead instead of continuing on the rest of the loop. To the left, a spur trail leads to another paved road, Bond Park Drive. Stay straight (southeast) and join the Pine Cone Trail.

The Pine Cone Trail (or "the little PCT," as I like to call it), like the Paw Paw Trail, is easy to follow. At most of the junctions, the trail is marked with blue arrows and signs that will help direct you back to the main trailhead or anywhere else you would like to go in the park from here. The Pine Cone Trail continues for 0.5 mile, crossing Bond Park Drive before climbing a steep hill, curving around to the right (south), and passing behind a row of homes on the left and two sports fields on the right. In 0.5 mile from the spot where you joined the Paw Paw Trail, you reach the intersection with the Black

Creek Greenway. Turn right (west) and continue onto a paved section of the Pine Cone Trail. Over the next 0.2 mile you pass behind two more sports fields on the right and pass by a spur trail on the right that leads to the Lazy Daze Playground. This is a great detour if you are walking with kids; otherwise stay straight (west) until you reach the trail junction with the Oxford Hunt Greenway and the Lake Trail. Turn right (north), and continue on the Pine Cone Trail for 0.2 mile, following along the lakeshore and climbing over several small hills, until you reach the main trailhead, kiosk, and the end of the trail. From here you can follow the spur trail behind the amphitheater to the parking lot at the Kiwanis shelter where you started.

Nearby Attractions

Hemlock Bluffs Nature Preserve (see page 66) is 4 miles to the west of Fred G. Bond Metro Park and has almost 4 miles of hiking trails. The trails in Hemlock Bluffs are slightly more challenging than the trails at Bond Park. The trails at Hemlock traverse small hills and lead to steep bluffs with views of Swift Creek below. The park is designated to protect clusters of eastern hemlocks on the north-facing bluffs and features a nature center geared toward young children.

Swift Creek Bluffs Nature Preserve (see page 111) is in southeast Cary, 6 miles southeast of Fred G. Bond Metro Park. The 23-acre preserve has a 1.2-mile trail that follows along Swift Creek to the bluffs.

Directions

From Raleigh follow Capital Boulevard/US 70 East for 2.2 miles and merge onto I-40 West toward Cary. Follow I-40 West for 7.2 miles. Take NC 54, Exit 290, toward Cary and follow NC 54 for 0.2 mile. Turn left onto Chapel Hill Road/NC 54 West and follow it 1.2 miles. Turn right onto northeast Maynard Road/NC 54 West and follow it 3.7 miles. Turn right onto High House Road and follow it 0.7 mile until you reach 801 High House Road and the entrance to Fred G. Bond Metro Park, on the left.

7

Harris Lake County Park

SCENERY: ★ ★ ★ ★
TRAIL CONDITION: ★ ★ ★ ★ ★
CHILDREN: ★ ★ ★ ★ ★
DIFFICULTY: ★ ★
SOLITUDE: ★

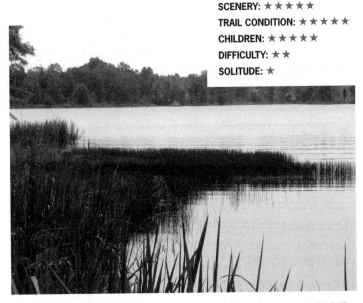

YOU WON'T HAVE A PROBLEM FINDING A GREAT VIEW OF HARRIS LAKE ON THE PENINSULA TRAIL.

GPS TRAILHEAD COORDINATES: N35° 37.209' W78° 55.643'

DISTANCE & CONFIGURATION: 4.5-mile loop

HIKING TIME: 2 hours

HIGHLIGHTS: Harris Lake

ELEVATION: 226' at trailhead to 265' at peak and 216' at lowest point

ACCESS: Daily, 8 a.m.–sunset; closed January 1, Thanksgiving, and December 24–25. Free.

MAPS: Online at wakegov.com/parks or at the park visitor center

FACILITIES: Restrooms, water fountains, disc golf course, volleyball course, picnic facilities and shelters, playground, open playing field, mountain bike trails, educational center, educational gardens, boat landing, canoe and kayak launch, and fishing pier

WHEELCHAIR ACCESS: None

COMMENTS: There are a variety of activities to explore at Harris Lake County Park. It is easy to make a day out of a visit. Consider bringing your mountain bike, fishing poles, canoes and kayaks, and other sports gear to get the most from this park's exceptional facilities.

CONTACTS: 919-387-4342; wakegov.com/parks

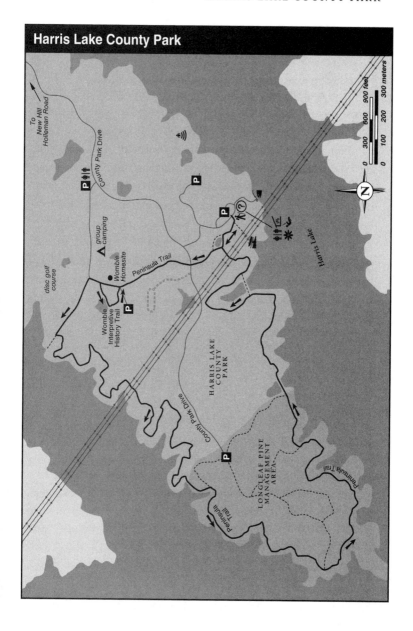

Harris Lake County Park

Overview

This 680-acre park is 23 miles southwest of Raleigh and 32 miles south of Durham.

This route combines the Peninsula Trail and the Womble Interpretive History Trail to create a 4.5-mile loop that ventures to the edge of the park's peninsula and explores the shore of Harris Lake. The Peninsula Trail travels through rich forests of hardwoods and oaks. Along the route you will learn about the history of the park through plaques along the Womble Interpretive History Trail, pass the historic Womble Homesite, and experience spectacular views of Harris Lake. Near the tip of the peninsula you will journey through thick stands of longleaf pines in the Longleaf Pine Management Area. Keep an eye out for the deer, turkeys, and a variety of waterfowl that inhabit the forests and surrounding Harris Lake. If the distance is intimidating—or just a little too much to handle for a hike with young children—there are many opportunities to make this route a shorter excursion by utilizing the many loop spur trails that you encounter near the beginning of the route.

Route Details

The Peninsula Trail starts from the parking lot, near the educational garden. A trailhead in the northwest corner of the lot is marked with a kiosk. Follow the path 100 feet until you a reach a junction in the trail. To the left a spur trail leads down toward the lake to the car-top boat launch. This is where visitors can launch johnboats, kayaks, canoes, and other small watercraft that do not require a trailer. Stay to the right (northwest) and follow the Peninsula Trail. About 300 feet later you reach a pond and another junction. Stay left (west) and follow the Peninsula Trail around the edge of the pond. Continue for 175 feet. You reach another junction here. Turn right (north), keeping the pond to your right, and continue on the Peninsula Trail for 150 feet, where you reach a split in the trail. To the right (east) the trail circles around the pond. Turn left (northwest) and stay on the

Peninsula Trail, heading toward the Womble Interpretive History Trail. Walk for 0.2 mile through the forest until you reach a junction with the Womble Interpretive History Trail. Turn left (west), staying on the Peninsula Trail and heading toward the Womble Homesite. After 0.1 mile you arrive at the Womble Homesite, where you can still see the relics of the home's foundation. There is also a trail junction with the other end of the Womble Interpretive History Trail here.

Before Progress Energy purchased this land, it was owned mostly by the Womble family, which had operated a small farm on this property since the 1700s. Little was known about the cultural history of the Womble family and the surrounding landowners until North Carolina State University graduate students Scott Bode and Sarah Nothstine conducted interviews with living heirs of the families who owned the land in this area. According to these interviews, the Womble family and the surrounding farms in the community raised livestock and grew mostly cotton, tobacco, sweet potatoes, and peanuts. Sugarcane was also grown for producing molasses. The families made their income by taking their crops and livestock to the markets in downtown Raleigh.

If you want to extend the length of this trail, you can turn left directly across from the Womble Homesite and explore the Womble Interpretive History Trail, a 0.1-mile loop that rejoins with Peninsula Trail 350 feet south of the homesite. Relics of small building sites, old farm tools, and interpretive plaques along the way add to the learning experience along this trail. At each interpretive station there is a phone number you can call on your cell phone to access information about the relics you are seeing. From the Womble Homesite, after living the Womble Interpretive History Trail, continue north for 125 feet until you reach another junction with a spur trail. Turn left (west) and head toward the disc golf course. After all those turns and junctions that were pretty hard to navigate, the trail gets very easy to follow from here.

Continue for 0.2 mile, following along the edge of the disc golf course to your right (north) and descending to the edge of Harris

Lake. From here the trail follows along the edge of Harris Lake. You get some spectacular views of the lake along the way, especially near the peninsula. Also, near the tip of the peninsula you will notice that the forest changes. You will see the hardwoods and oaks disappear and find yourself in a forest of pine trees. Here you are walking through the Longleaf Pine Management Area. Along this section of trail, on the southern side of the lake, several spur trails lead off to your left. Just stay to the right and keep on the Peninsula Trail. Follow the trail for 3.4 miles around the lake until you reach the car-top boat-launch spur trail again. Stay left (east) and follow the Peninsula Trail back to the parking lot and trailhead where you started.

Nearby Attractions

The 174-acre Historic Yates Mill County Park (see page 82) is 21 miles northeast of Harris Lake County Park. The park has more than 2 miles of hiking trails that explore the surrounding wetlands and forests and circle around a 20-acre pond fed by Steep Hill Creek and its tributaries. The main feature of the park is Yates Mill, a masterfully restored 18th-century water-powered gristmill. Built by Samuel Pearson sometime between 1763 and 1778, the gristmill is the only fully operational water-powered gristmill in Wake County.

Raven Rock State Park (see pages 93 and 99) has more than 11 miles of hiking trails and 10 miles of horseback-riding bridle trails on 4,667 acres of land. Discover the park's intriguing rock formations along miles of trails that explore the shore of the Cape Fear River and the surrounding beautiful landscape.

Directions

From Raleigh, follow Capital Boulevard/US 70 East for 2.3 miles. Merge onto I-40 West and follow it toward Cary for 4.8 miles. Take the I-440 East exit, Exit 293, toward Raleigh/Cary/Wake Forest and follow it 0.9 mile. Merge onto US 1 South via Exit 293A toward Cary/Asheboro and follow it 13 miles. Take Exit 89 toward New Hill/Jordan

Lake and follow the road 0.9 mile. Turn left onto New Hill Holleman Road and follow it 2.9 miles. Turn right onto County Park Drive, and after 0.1 mile you will reach Harris Lake County Park, on the right. If you reach the end of County Park Drive, you've gone too far.

From Durham, take the Fayetteville Street exit ramp onto NC 147 South and follow it 6.7 miles. To avoid the toll section of NC 147, merge onto I-40 East via Exit 5A on the left, toward RDU Airport/Raleigh, and follow it 13.3 miles. Take the I-440 East exit, Exit 293, toward Cary/Wake Forest, and after 0.3 mile merge onto US 1 South via Exit 293A toward Cary/Asheboro and follow it 12.8 miles. Take Exit 89 toward New Hill/Jordan Lake and follow it 0.2 mile. Turn left onto New Hill Holleman Road and follow it 2.9 miles. Turn right onto County Park Drive and continue 0.1 mile until you reach Harris Lake County Park, on the right. If you reach the end of County Park Drive, you've gone too far.

Hemlock Bluffs
Nature Preserve

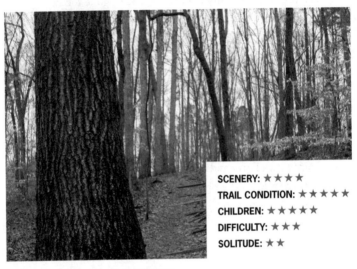

SCENERY: ★ ★ ★ ★
TRAIL CONDITION: ★ ★ ★ ★ ★
CHILDREN: ★ ★ ★ ★ ★
DIFFICULTY: ★ ★ ★
SOLITUDE: ★ ★

A FOREST SCENE AT HEMLOCK BLUFFS

GPS TRAILHEAD COORDINATES: N35° 43.411' W78° 47.008'

DISTANCE & CONFIGURATION: 1.4-mile loop

HIKING TIME: 1 hour

HIGHLIGHTS: Hemlock Bluffs, bluff overlooks, Swift Creek, nature center, and a children's garden

ELEVATION: 417' at trailhead to 357' at lowest point

ACCESS: Park: Daily, 9 a.m.–sunset. Nature center: May–September, daily, 9 a.m.–7 p.m.; October–April, daily, 9 a.m.–5 p.m.; free

MAPS: At the trailhead kiosk and at the nature center

FACILITIES: Water fountains and restrooms

WHEELCHAIR ACCESS: Only at the nature center

COMMENTS: The trails are very popular and great for running. Dogs are welcome in the preserve but must be kept on a leash. If you want to visit the preserve when it is less crowded, avoid weekends and holidays. The decks at the bluff overlooks have railings and are very safe; nevertheless, keep an eye on kids and don't let them wander too far afield. The bluffs are steep and can pose a safety risk to children in some areas along the trail.

CONTACTS: 919-387-5980; townofcary.org

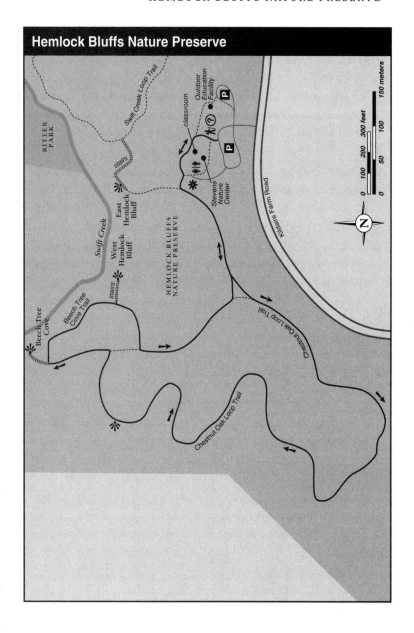

Hemlock Bluffs Nature Preserve

Overview

This is a very enjoyable walk through the ridges and ravines of Cary's upland forest.

Cary is 10 miles west of downtown Raleigh, and the 150-acre Hemlock Bluffs Nature Preserve has more than 3 miles of trails that traverse a hilly area of forest atop a steep bluff with views of Swift Creek below. This 1.3-mile walk combines the Chestnut Oak Loop and Beech Tree Cove Trails and leads through several sections of eastern hemlocks along the north-facing bluffs. The bluffs provide a cool, moist microclimate in which the hemlocks thrive. The trail is very well maintained, and the trail surfaces are covered with mulch, which provides a very soft and cushiony feel that is especially welcome for runners and hikers who have knee troubles. The nature center at the trailhead is mostly geared toward children, and a children's garden is displayed at the beginning of the trail behind the nature center. Along the trail you will see bird boxes of varying sizes, the largest of them for barred owls.

Route Details

Park at the Stevens Nature Center. The trail starts from the kiosk in front of the nature center. Follow the paved stone spur trail uphill to the nature center, passing the large, covered pavilion on the right, until you reach a trail junction. Turn left (east) onto the paved trail and walk toward the overlooks, passing the children's garden on the left. Continue 100 feet until you reach the wooden arbor on the right. Turn right (west) onto the 7-foot-wide, mulch-covered trail. The trail is very well maintained—some of the best trail maintenance I have seen in Raleigh. It is very easy to follow, and signs mark most of the trail junctions, which makes this a great trail for families and young kids.

After 80 feet you reach another trail junction. Turn left (southwest) onto the Chestnut Oak Loop Trail and toward the West Hemlock Bluffs. Continue for 0.1 mile until you reach a split in the trail. Stay to the left (south) and continue on the mulch-covered trail. After

300 feet, veer to the right and pass a spur trail leading to a small maintenance area. Continue toward the Chestnut Oak Overlook for 0.6 mile. The trail gently descends to the creek and follows alongside a small stream before passing over some small hills and reaching the small wooden overlook deck. Chestnut Oak Overlook is on the left side of the trail and overlooks a bluff and a small winding stream below. From here the trail climbs gently uphill and crosses a short wooden footbridge before reaching a trail junction after 300 feet. Turn left (north) and continue toward Beech Tree Cove Overlook.

The trail descends a small hill and after 250 feet reaches the spur trail to the Beech Tree Cove Overlook. If you stay straight (north), the spur trail leads down a wooden staircase to the overlook of the bluffs and Swift Creek. Turn right (east) and continue toward the West Hemlock Bluffs Overlook. Climb the steep hill that provides 33 feet of elevation gain over the next 300 feet and reach a trail junction. Turn left (east) onto the spur trail and walk to the West Hemlock Bluffs Overlook with views of the bluffs and Swift Creek winding through the forest below. In the forest, on the north side of the overlook deck, you will see several eastern hemlock trees along the bluff's edge. These are some of the very trees that this preserve has been established to protect. Eastern hemlocks are exceptionally rare in this part of the United States, as eastern North Carolina is just on the edge of their habitat range. These tall trees usually grow to be more than 100 feet tall and have a lifespan of more than 500 years.

After enjoying the overlook deck, turn around and continue uphill to the main trail, which heads south toward the nature center. After 0.1 mile, you reach a trail junction. Turn left (south), following the signs that direct you toward the park entrance. The trail along this section is very easy to follow and well maintained, and after 300 feet you reach a split in the trail. Turn left (east) and continue heading toward the park entrance. The trail climbs uphill for 0.2 mile, passing the nature center on the right and reaching the kiosk, trailhead, and the end of the trail.

Nearby Attractions

There is another, shorter 0.8-mile loop in the Hemlock Bluffs Nature Preserve called the Swift Creek Loop Trail. It offers views of more of the protected hemlock trees from the west bluffs. There is an extensive network of boardwalks along this shorter trail and more than 100 stairs to climb, so be prepared for more elevation gain on this trail than on the Chestnut Oak Loop Trail.

Swift Creek Bluffs Nature Preserve (see page 111) is 4 miles to the east of Hemlock Bluffs. The 23-acre preserve has a 1.2-mile trail that follows along Swift Creek to the bluffs. Fred G. Bond Metro Park (see pages 50 and 55) is 7 miles to the north of Hemlock Bluffs. The metro park is 310 acres and offers more than 4 miles of walking and biking trails that center on Bond Lake. The Black Creek Greenway, Oxford Hunt Greenway, and White Oak Greenway all intersect at Fred G. Bond Metro Park.

Directions

From Raleigh take I-440 toward Cary, and then take US 1 South toward Sanford. Take Exit 98A/Tryon Road. Go to the third stoplight and turn right onto Kildaire Farm Road. Go through two stoplights (past Lochmere Golf Course and a shopping center on your left). You will cross a bridge and round a curve. Look for a driveway on the right. A blue entrance sign will be visible as you turn into the parking lot.

From Chapel Hill or other points west, take I-40 East to Exit 293A. This will put you on US 1 South/US 64 West. Take Exit 98A/ Tryon Road. Go to the third stoplight and turn right onto Kildaire Farm Road. Go through two stoplights (past Lochmere Golf Course and a shopping center on your left). You will cross a bridge and round a curve. Look for a driveway on the right. A blue entrance sign will be visible as you turn into the parking lot.

Historic Oak View County Park

SCENERY: ★ ★ ★ ★ ★
TRAIL CONDITION: ★ ★ ★ ★ ★
CHILDREN: ★ ★ ★ ★ ★
DIFFICULTY: ★ ★
SOLITUDE: ★ ★

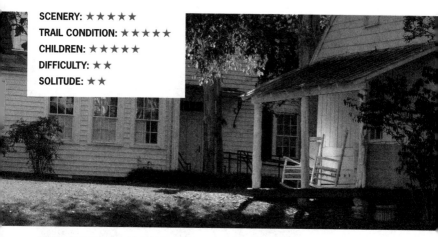

STEP BACK IN TIME AT THE HISTORIC OAK VIEW COUNTY PARK.

GPS TRAILHEAD COORDINATES: N35° 46.248' W78° 34.326'

DISTANCE & CONFIGURATION: 0.3-mile balloon

HIKING TIME: 1 hour

HIGHLIGHTS: Farm History Center, historic barn, main farmhouse, and cotton museum

ELEVATION: 284' at trailhead to 298' at peak

ACCESS: Monday–Saturday, 8:30 a.m.–5 p.m.; Sunday 1–5 p.m.; closed January 1, Thanksgiving, and December 24–25; main farmhouse closed Monday; free

MAPS: At the Farm History Center

FACILITIES: Restrooms, water fountains, and picnic area

WHEELCHAIR ACCESS: Yes

COMMENTS: The surrounding grounds and the pecan grove to the east are also part of the park and open to the public. Feel free to explore the land around the main house. The animals in the livestock area in the west area of the park are very friendly, so pet the goats if you want. The park is very popular with school groups and families with children, so it can be quite busy and often loud 11 a.m.–3 p.m. If you want to explore the park in peace, the best time to go is in the morning and the evening during weekdays, before and after the school groups have usually left. Dogs are allowed in the park, but they must be kept on a leash no longer than 6 feet at all times. No bikes are allowed on the paths.

CONTACTS: 919-250-1013; wakegov.com/parks

Historic Oak View County Park

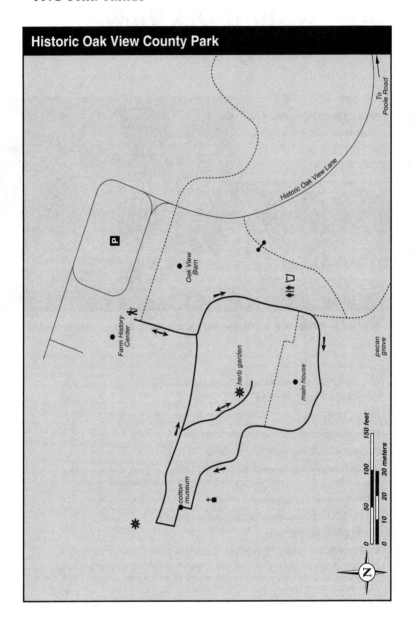

Overview

Historic Oak View County Park is 5 miles east of downtown Raleigh, and it is definitely worth the trip. The incredibly preserved 27-acre farmstead can be explored along more than a mile of paths. This trail starts at the Farm History Center, a museum with exhibits for adults and children that tell the story of farming in North Carolina. From the Farm History Center you follow an easy and level path that is mostly paved with cobblestone and brick. You pass a historic barn, the main farmhouse, and the water tower and head to the oldest building on the property, a plank kitchen with an herb garden growing outside. From the garden you pass a cemetery, where many of the farm owners through the years were laid to rest, and continue to the cotton museum, with a fine example of a cotton field growing out front. From here the trail circles around and returns to the trailhead in front of the Farm History Center.

Route Details

When you set foot on this land, it's hard to imagine that the surrounding 28 acres were purchased for only $135, and today you can explore them for free. Follow Historic Oak View Lane to the parking lot behind the Farm History Center, where you can get a great map, artfully illustrated by Patrick Pleasants. At the Farm History Center you can explore exhibits that describe North Carolina's long and mostly successful agricultural history. At the Farmer's Corner, you will find exhibits specially designed and interpreted for children.

After stepping out of the Farm History Center, you find the trailhead to your right. Follow the pebble path to the redbrick path and turn left (east) toward the main house. You quickly come to Oak View Barn. The barn was built circa 1900, and today it is used for school programs, for private functions, and as a home for Boyd and Quint, the two nicest Nubian goats you are ever likely to meet. During operating hours the goats are usually found hanging around the edge of the fenced-in area just beside the barn, and you're welcome to pet them. Next to the barn, in what used to be the carriage house, are restrooms, where you can get a sip of water from the water fountains and wash your hands after petting the goats.

The carriage house was also built around 1900. In the 1940s it was converted into a two-car garage, but it originally housed the farm's carriage, and, yes, it was the kind pulled by horses. After passing the carriage house, you reach a split in the trail. If you stay straight (south), the path continues away from the farmstead area and enters into the pecan grove. After you're done exploring the farm, the trail through the pecan grove is a great place to stroll if you're not yet tired of walking. In the meantime, turn right (west) and follow the redbrick path to the main farmhouse. The farmhouse was built by the first owner of the property, Benton S. D. Williams, in 1855 and remodeled in the 1940s by J. Gregory Poole Sr. Except on Tuesdays the two-story Greek Revival home is open for visitors to explore, so just open the door and venture inside.

The paved path curves around the side of the main house until it reaches an intersection with another paved path. Turn left (northwest) toward the cotton museum. You pass the cemetery on the left. Williams—along with many other farm owners and their family members, who worked hard to farm the surrounding land for many generations—is laid to rest in this cemetery. Continue to the cotton museum directly in front of you. The museum and its exhibits on growing cotton are open for exploration. You follow the exhibits through the opening in the building and out the back door, where you find a carriage holding a cotton bale. To the right is the cotton field.

Follow the path around the cotton museum and past the cotton field and continue to the garden and plank kitchen. A small path leads through the small herb garden and into the plank kitchen, the oldest building on the property, constructed around 1825. The door is always open, and a collection of cooking tools that were used on the farm during earlier times is on display inside. From here, turn around and follow the path through the herb garden. Once you reach the main paved path, turn right (southeast) and follow the paved path for 450 feet back to the trailhead, Farm History Center, and parking lot.

Nearby Attractions

Clemmons Educational State Forest (see page 32), with more than 6 miles of hiking trails, is 10 miles to the north of Historic Oak View County Park. Clemmons is an education park geared toward children, with trails that traverse a landscape of rolling hills and creeks. A loop trail circles a pond in the north section of the park, and trails with an impressive collection of interpretive kiosks explore the natural history of the forest and give insight into how the forest is managed and harvested.

Downtown Raleigh (see page 44) is just 5 miles to the west of the Historic Oak View County Park. You can explore downtown's business district along Fayetteville Street, take a tour of the State Capitol, or just stroll to the quaint City Market and stop in for a coffee-sipping experience at a historic café. Also downtown is the historic neighborhood of Oakwood (see page 76) and the Mordecai Historic Park, both with the best examples of 19th-century homes, and some of the finest examples of Victorian architecture in the South. On the southeastern border of the Oakwood neighborhood, you will find the governor's mansion, and it is definitely worth touring the home's lavish interior, which may be enough to convince anyone to start politicking.

Directions

From Raleigh, take I-440 East toward Rocky Mount and follow it 3.7 miles. Take the Poole Road exit, Exit 15, and turn left onto Poole Road. Follow Poole Road 0.4 mile. Turn left onto Carya Drive and follow it 0.1 mile. Historic Oak View County Park will be on the left.

10

Historic Oakwood Neighborhood Walk

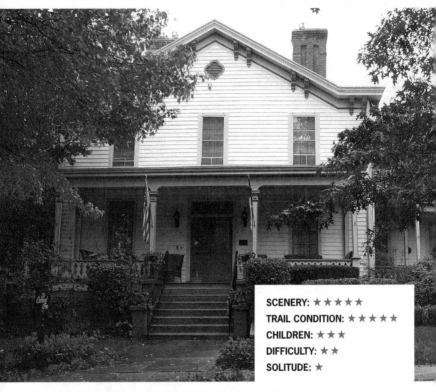

SCENERY: ★ ★ ★ ★ ★
TRAIL CONDITION: ★ ★ ★ ★ ★
CHILDREN: ★ ★ ★
DIFFICULTY: ★ ★
SOLITUDE: ★

TAKE A TOUR THROUGH ONE OF THE MOST WELL-PRESERVED HISTORIC NEIGHBORHOODS IN RALEIGH.

GPS TRAILHEAD COORDINATES: N35° 46.943' W78° 38.091'

DISTANCE & CONFIGURATION: 2.0-mile double loop

HIKING TIME: 1.5 hours

HIGHLIGHTS: Governor's mansion, historic homes, and Oakwood Inn Bed and Breakfast

ELEVATION: 335' at trailhead to 281' at lowest point

ACCESS: 24/7; free

MAPS: Online at historicoakwood.org and at the Raleigh Visitor Information Center (500 Fayetteville St.)

FACILITIES: None

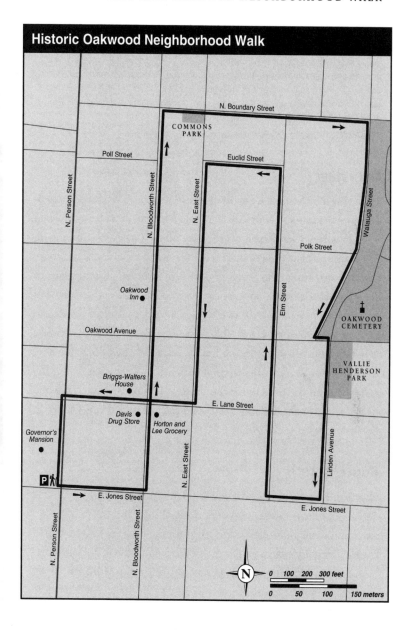

WHEELCHAIR ACCESS: Yes, paved sidewalks are throughout the area.

COMMENTS: The busiest time of the year to explore the Oakwood neighborhood is during the spring and fall, when the weather is tolerably cool. Adding a tour of the governor's mansion can add a lot to a trip to the neighborhood. Oakwood is a residential and business district, and therefore dogs are welcome as long as they are on a leash no longer than 6 feet. Please be respectful of the residents in the neighborhood and treat this walk as if you are walking through your own neighborhood.

CONTACTS: 919-833-1120; historicoakwood.org

Overview

Listed on the National Register of Historic Places, Oakwood is one of the finest examples of late-1800s development in downtown Raleigh. This downtown walk explores the core of the classic neighborhood. The walk starts at the governor's mansion and follows a short route that winds through the center of the neighborhood, passing many of the key historic homes in the neighborhood as well as the Oakwood Inn Bed and Breakfast, Oakwood Cemetery, and houses developed by Colonel Jonathan Heck. This charming walk through Oakwood can only be made better by adding a tour of the governor's mansion to the schedule. Or visit the neighborhood in December, when the residents and the Society for the Preservation of Historic Oakwood hold their annual candlelight tour, and the interiors of the Oakwood homes are open to the public.

Route Details

The first houses in the Oakwood neighborhood were built in the 1870s. Then the streets here were made of dirt, and the people who lived in the neighborhood could tell stories of how they remembered the day, only five years earlier in 1865, when General William Sherman marched into town and set up camp here. The Mordecai family owned the land at that time, and when they began to sell small lots to a mixture of upper-middle-class and working-class residents of Raleigh, homes were constructed in Queen Anne and Second Empire styles, but mostly in the Carolina vernacular style.

After World War II, the neighborhood began to fall into decline, and most of the wealthy residents moved to more-fashionable neighborhoods. Dilapidation set in, and, unbelievably, in 1972 the city of Raleigh had slated part of the neighborhood to be destroyed so that the North to South Expressway could be built. The Society for the Preservation of Historic Oakwood was formed, and through outreach programs such as annual candlelight tours and action through local government, the society saved the neighborhood from destruction and began a restoration campaign that would eventually find the Oakwood neighborhood listed in 1972 as Raleigh's first federally designated historic district.

This walk through Oakwood begins at the governor's mansion, on the corner of East Jones and North Person Streets. The home is the state of North Carolina's third gubernatorial mansion, and most of the materials used to build the mansion were gathered from around the state, including the clay bricks from Wake County and the heart pine and oak brought in from all over the state. The mansion is very ornate and elaborately appointed with antique furnishings. Tours can be scheduled by contacting the Capital Area Visitor Center and are highly recommended as part of your visit to the historic Oakwood neighborhood.

Start walking east on East Jones Street toward the 200 block. Walk one block and turn left (north) onto North Bloodworth Street. On the northeast side of the 200 block along Bloodworth Street, you enter into the historic business district of Oakwood, which includes the preserved Horton and Lee Grocery building, at 222 Bloodworth St., and the Davis Drug Store building, at 225 Bloodworth St. The oldest section of the Davis building is the corner building, constructed in 1913.

Continue on North Bloodworth Street for 0.2 mile, crossing East Lane Street and Oakwood Avenue, until you arrive at the Oakwood Inn Bed and Breakfast. The Oakwood Inn, Raleigh's first bed-and-breakfast, at 411 N. Bloodworth St., was built in 1871 and is historically known as the Strong-Stronach House. In fact, it wasn't until 1983 that the home became a business and was opened as the Oakwood Inn. The home was originally built in the 1880s by Thomas H. Briggs for then–state legislator George Strong, a grocer and former Confederate major. It is considered the best example of Italianate-style architecture in the Oakwood neighborhood.

Continue north on North Bloodworth Street for 0.2 mile until you reach North Boundary Street. Turn right (east) onto North Boundary Street. Continue for 0.2 mile, passing the Oakwood Commons Park and playground on the right, and then turn right (south) onto Watauga Street. Along the right (west) side of the road is Oakwood Green, a section of newer development, and to the left (east) side of the road is the Oakwood Cemetery, a 102-acre historical burial ground that includes a special 2-acre section, where 1,390 Confederate soldiers are laid to rest. The cemetery acts as the eastern border of the Oakwood Historic District.

Continue another 0.2 mile, passing the cemetery, until you reach Oakwood Avenue. Turn left (east) onto Oakwood Avenue and walk for just 80 feet before turning right (south) onto Linden Avenue. On the northeast corner of Oakwood Avenue and Linden Avenue is Vallie Henderson Park, a small park established in the memory of the Oakwood Garden Club's founder. Continue south on Linden Avenue for 0.2 mile and turn right (west) onto East Jones Street. Walk one block and turn right (north) onto Elm Street. Continue for four blocks or 0.3 mile, passing through Pullentown, a section of the neighborhood built by philanthropist and developer Richard Stanhope Pullen, and then turn left (west) onto Euclid Street.

Walk one block and turn left (south) onto North East Street. Continue for three blocks or 0.2 mile and turn right (west) onto East Lane Street. Walk for two blocks or 0.1 mile, passing the Briggs-Walters House at 321 E. Lane St. Thomas H. Briggs built this home in 1895 on the site where, on April 13, 1865, General Judson Kilpatrick hanged a soldier known only as Lieutenant Walsh for firing on him after the city had surrendered. After walking these two blocks, you reach the northeast corner of the governor's mansion and the end of the Oakwood historic neighborhood walk.

Nearby Attractions

The Mordecai Historic Park (919-857-4364), at 1 Mimosa St., is just 1 mile north of Oakwood and makes a great addition to a day of touring historic homes and neighborhoods in Raleigh. Admission to the park, which includes a 1-hour tour, is just $5 for adults and $3 for children and seniors. Tours are offered Tuesday–Sunday, but the park grounds are open daily, sunrise–sunset.

Located in downtown Raleigh (see page 44), Oakwood is close to downtown Raleigh's business district, where you will find plenty of restaurants, shopping, and accommodations to explore. Recommended is the City Market between Martin Street and Davie Street, one block east of Wilmington Street. Also near downtown Raleigh is North Carolina State University, 14 miles west of Oakwood.

Directions

Oakwood is in downtown Raleigh. From the visitor center at the Raleigh Marriott City Center, at 500 Fayetteville St., start out going north on Fayetteville Street toward Hanover Square and follow the street 0.4 mile. Turn right onto East Morgan Street and follow it 0.3 mile. Turn left onto North Person Street and continue 0.2 mile. Turn left onto East Lane Street and follow it 0.1 mile. The governor's mansion will be on your left, at 200 E. Lane St.

11

Historic Yates Mill County Park

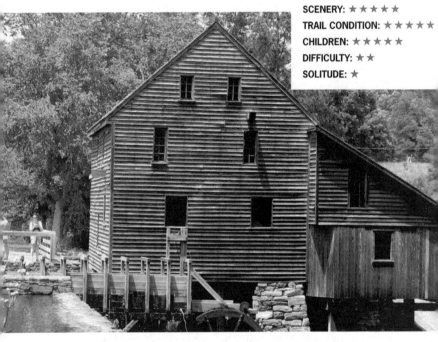

SCENERY: ★ ★ ★ ★ ★
TRAIL CONDITION: ★ ★ ★ ★ ★
CHILDREN: ★ ★ ★ ★ ★
DIFFICULTY: ★ ★
SOLITUDE: ★

HIKERS CAN WALK RIGHT UP BESIDE THE HISTORIC YATES MILL.

GPS TRAILHEAD COORDINATES: N35° 43.188' W78° 41.211'

DISTANCE & CONFIGURATION: 1.3-mile loop

HIKING TIME: 1 hour

HIGHLIGHTS: Yates Mill

ELEVATION: 302' at trailhead to 357' at peak

ACCESS: Grounds: Daily, 8 a.m.–sunset. Center: Daily, 8:30 a.m.–5 p.m.
Closed January 1, Thanksgiving, and December 24–25. Free.

MAPS: Online at wakegov.com/parks and at the park visitor center

FACILITIES: Restrooms and water fountains

WHEELCHAIR ACCESS: None

COMMENTS: The park is very popular with children and families. Avoid crowds by visiting
early in the morning and after 3 p.m. on weekdays.

CONTACTS: 919-856-6675; wakegov.com/parks

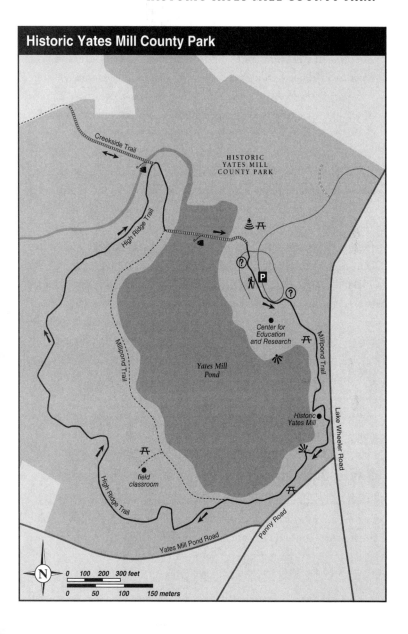

Historic Yates Mill County Park

Overview

The 174-acre Historic Yates Mill County Park is 6 miles south of downtown Raleigh, and it features the masterfully restored water-powered 18th-century Yates Mill. The park has more than 2 miles of hiking trails, which circle around a 20-acre pond fed by Steep Hill Creek and its tributaries. The trails explore the park's surrounding wetlands and forests. This route starts at the park's main facility, the A. E. Finley Center for Education, and follows the Millpond Trail across an impressive wooden boardwalk spanning the pond, with viewing scopes and benches that offers impressive views of the water. The trail then continues north and merges with the Creekside Trail for a 1-mile hike through the park's wetlands and forests, but don't worry—boardwalks keep your feet dry when you pass through the wetland areas. At the end of the Creekside Trail you turn around, backtrack on the Creekside Trail, and then follow the High Ridge Trail, which traverses the ridges above the pond, passing through mixed old field pine and hardwood forests. The High Ridge Trail rejoins with the Millpond Trail, which follows the pond shore, passing an observation deck of the water-powered mill at the end of the hike. You then return to the A. E. Finley Center for Education, where you will find much-welcomed rocking chairs on the porch to relax and enjoy views of the serene pond and the surrounding landscape.

Route Details

The A. E. Finley Center for Education and Research includes two classrooms, an auditorium, and an exhibit hall. One of the most popular areas of the center is the porch with rocking chairs. The center closes at 5 p.m. every day, but the restrooms are open daily, 8 a.m.–sunset.

A kiosk at the south end of the parking lot, in front of the A. E. Finley Center for Education and Research, marks the start of the Millpond Trail. Three feet from the start of the trail, you pass picnic tables. The 4-foot-wide gravel path is lined with stones and follows along the edge of the lakeshore. Follow the gravel path for 0.1 mile, crossing a wooden bridge that spans a small creek, and follow stone steps that lead up to the front of the historic Yates Mill.

The water-powered Yates Mill provided the vital service of grinding corn and wheat into meal and flour in Wake County for more than 200 years. At one time there were more than 70 gristmills in Wake County, and Yates Mill is the only one that is still in operation. Before grocery and convenient stores, the gristmill acted as a gathering place for rural communities that were scattered and separated by long distances. Today Yates Mill Pond is used for swimming and fishing.

Samuel Pearson built the mill sometime between 1763 and 1778; the Revolutionary War interrupted the land survey that would have recorded the actual date the mill was built. The mill was passed to Simon Pearson, one of Pearson's sons, after his death, and debts owed to the bank forced the son to sell the mill and the 340 acres he inherited in a sheriff's sale. The mill passed through many owners over the next 200 years and operated until the 1950s, when it closed for a lack of business. The University of North Carolina acquired the land in 1963 for use as experimental farms and demonstration fields. In 1989, the Yates Mill Associates was formed, with its goal being to preserve and restore the dilapidated mill. The Wake County Board of Commissioners approved the park's master plan in 1997, and in 2006 construction of the park's visitor center was completed. The park finally opened to the public May 20, 2006, almost 250 years after the mill was first constructed. Mill tours are available March–November, and on the third weekend of each month, the park offers corn-grinding demonstrations by costumed interpreters.

Follow the dirt road around the left side of Yates Mill. After 0.1 mile you reach a junction with the High Ridge Trail. If you want to make this route shorter, just stay straight and follow the Millpond Trail around the edge of the pond, circling back to the visitor center. For a longer hike, turn left (west) and follow the High Ridge Trail, which ascends to a ridge above the lake. Walk on the High Ridge Trail for 0.6 mile until you reach a junction with the Creekside Trail. To further extend this route, you can hike the Creekside Trail to its end a mile away and then turn around and hike back. At the very least, I recommended hiking the first 400 feet of this Creekside Trail. Turn left (northwest) and follow the Creekside Trail across the boardwalk that explores a wetland area. At the end of the boardwalk you can continue for the next mile through the forest if you like, which will add 2 more miles to your hike. For the route featured here, head back across the boardwalk (southeast) toward the Millpond Trail.

After crossing the boardwalk, you reach the junction with the High Ridge Trail. Stay straight (southeast) and continue on the High Ridge Trail toward the Millpond Trail. After 350 feet, you reach a split in the trail where the High Ridge Trail runs into the Millpond Trail. Stay to the left (east) and follow the Millpond Trail across the boardwalk. You have a great view of the pond from here. After 500 feet from the junction with the High Ridge Trail, you will reach the north side of the parking lot where you started. The visitor center is straight ahead, to the south.

Nearby Attractions

Lake Johnson (see page 88) has more than 5 miles of hiking trails, as well as 300 acres of parkland that surround it. The lake is also great for fishing, and here you can catch largemouth bass, shellcracker, crappie, bream, catfish, and carp. Lake Johnson is 5 miles north of Historic Yates Mill County Park.

Seven miles west of Historic Yates Mill County Park is Hemlock Bluffs Nature Preserve (see page 66), which offers nearly 3 miles of hiking trails through a very well-maintained and beautiful park and was established to protect rare eastern hemlock trees on the north-facing bluffs. The park has an impressive 3,700-square-foot nature center with various programs geared toward children, as well as restrooms, water fountains, a gift shop, and a lecture hall.

Fred G. Bond Metro Park (see pages 50 and 55) is 13 miles northwest of Historic Yates Mill County Park. The metro park covers

310 acres and offers more than 4 miles of walking and biking trails that center on Bond Lake. The park is also the intersection for several of Cary's greenway trails, including the Black Creek Greenway, Oxford Hunt Greenway, and White Oak Greenway.

The 680-acre Harris Lake County Park (see page 60) is 19 miles south of Historic Yates Mill County Park in New Hill, North Carolina. The park has more than 7 miles of hiking trails, more than 10 miles of mountain-biking trails, a disc golf course, and boat ramps into the surrounding Harris Lake. Most of the hiking trails explore the shore of the lake peninsula and traverse longleaf pine forests.

Only 19 miles to the west is Jordan Lake State Park, with more than 22 miles of hiking trails that are spread out around Jordan Lake at the Ebenezer Church Recreation Area (see page 175), New Hope Overlook (see page 169), Vista Point, Seaforth (see page 180), Parker's Creek, Crosswinds Campground, and Poplar Point Campground.

Directions

From downtown Raleigh, start out going east on Capital Boulevard/US 70 East, and follow it 0.9 mile. Turn right onto West Lenoir Street and follow it 0.2 mile. Take the second left onto South Saunders Street and follow it 0.3 mile. Turn right onto Lake Wheeler Road and follow it 4.3 miles. The entrance to Historic Yates Mill County Park is on the right. If you reach Penny Road, you've gone too far.

From Durham, take I-40 East via Exit 5A toward RDU Airport/Raleigh and follow it 15.9 miles. Take the Gorman Street exit, Exit 295, and turn right onto Gorman Street, following it 0.1 mile. Take the first left onto Tryon Road and follow it 1.3 miles. Turn right onto Lake Wheeler Road and follow it 1.8 miles. The entrance to Historic Yates Mill County Park is on the right. If you reach Penny Road, you've gone too far.

12

Lake Johnson Park:
East Loop of Walnut Creek Trail

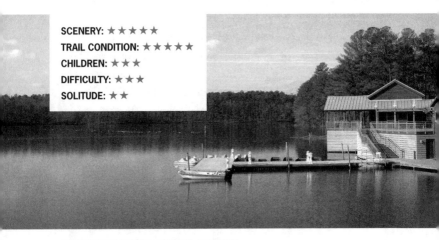

SCENERY: ★ ★ ★ ★ ★
TRAIL CONDITION: ★ ★ ★ ★ ★
CHILDREN: ★ ★ ★
DIFFICULTY: ★ ★ ★
SOLITUDE: ★ ★

AN EXCELLENT VISTA OF LAKE JOHNSON

GPS TRAILHEAD COORDINATES: N35° 45.749' W78° 42.845'

DISTANCE & CONFIGURATION: 2.8-mile loop

HIKING TIME: 2 hours

HIGHLIGHTS: Lake Johnson and Magnolia Cottage

ELEVATION: 350' at trailhead to 422' at peak

ACCESS: April–September: Daily, sunrise–sunset. October–March: Tuesday–Sunday, sunrise–sunset; closed January 1, Martin Luther King Jr. Day, Thanksgiving, and December 24–25. Free.

MAPS: Online at raleighnc.gov, at the park boathouse, or at the trailhead kiosk

FACILITIES: Boathouse, concessions, restrooms, picnic tables and pavilions, playground, and water fountains

WHEELCHAIR ACCESS: Yes, at the park and the east loop (but not the west loop) of the Walnut Creek Trail.

COMMENTS: The paved east loop of the Walnut Creek Trail is great for running and biking. To avoid colliding with bikers, stay alert, especially when walking around some of the blind curves at the base of hills, where bikers can be coming down the hill very fast. Dogs are welcome inside the park as well, as long as they are well behaved and kept on leashes no more than 6 feet long. To avoid crowds, enjoy the park during weekday work hours. Weekends, holidays, and mornings can be especially busy times.

CONTACTS: 919-233-2121; raleighnc.gov

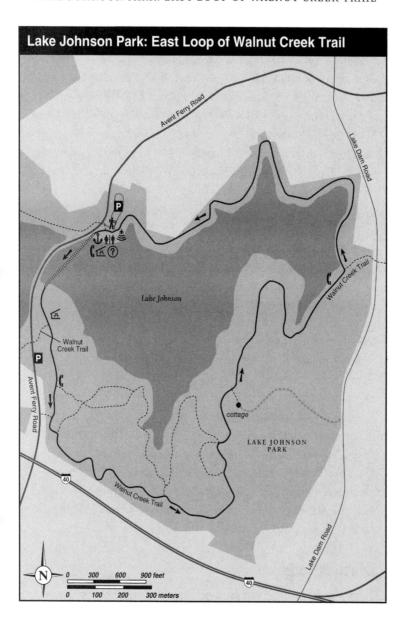

Lake Johnson Park: East Loop of Walnut Creek Trail

Overview

Lake Johnson Park is in west Raleigh, 6 miles or a 12-minute drive from downtown. The park centers on Lake Johnson, and the main trail in the park, the Lake Johnson segment of Walnut Creek Trail, circles the shore of the lake. The unpaved west loop of Walnut Creek Trail is less used and great for running if you are interested in a more cushioned surface to run on or enjoy hiking in more of a wilderness setting. The east loop of the Walnut Creek Trail, the longer of the two loops, is a 2.8-mile paved trail that starts at the boathouse and begins by crossing over a narrow section of Lake Johnson via a long, elevated boardwalk. The boardwalk is a nice start to the trail and offers great views of the lake, as well as an opportunity to fish if you bring your pole and tackle along. While the entire east loop may be a bit long for very young children, the walk onto the elevated boardwalk with views of the lake is recommended.

From here the east loop circles the lake, staying close to the lakeshore, and ventures through the forest that borders Lake Johnson. At times the trail passes behind homes whose backyards sit close to the lakeshore, and several spur trails lead into the nearby neighborhoods, connecting the neighborhoods with the greenway system around the lake. On the east side of the lake you pass Magnolia Cottage, a one-level structure nestled in the forest on the lakeshore. The cottage can be rented for special events. After passing Magnolia Cottage, you cross a small arched bridge that leads to a paved berm with open views of the lake to the west. The trail circles the perimeter of the lake's north shore before returning to the parking lot and trailhead.

Route Details

Enter via the park's main entrance and park at the lot in front of the boathouse. Both the unpaved west loop and the paved east loop of the Walnut Creek Trail begin at the west side of the boathouse. If you're facing the boathouse, the trail starts to the right of the building, where the raised walkway crosses the lake. Follow the elevated boardwalk, which offers excellent views of the lake, for 0.2 mile to the south shore of Lake Johnson. You can fish from the elevated boardwalk. Largemouth bass, shellcracker, crappie, bream, catfish, and carp are all found in Lake Johnson.

After crossing the boardwalk, the Walnut Creek Trail becomes paved and gently climbs to a split in the trail. To the right (west), the trail crosses the park's main road and continues to the unpaved west loop. However, stay straight (south) on the east loop. Continue 0.1 mile until you reach a split in the trail. To the right (west), a spur trail leads to a parking lot along the park's main road. To the left (east), a short spur trail leads to a scenic overlook with nice views of the lake. Stay straight (south) and continue on the east loop. Along this next section, several spur trails on the right side of the trail lead into a neighborhood, but stay straight on the paved east loop.

The trail becomes a little more challenging as it climbs a series of small hills during the next 0.6 mile. The trail really winds through the forest on this section, and there can be some blind turns, so watch out for bikers racing down some of the steep hills. The trail veers away from the lakeshore and passes the southern arm of the lake before turning sharply to the left (north) and reaching a trail junction. You can go either way at this junction because both spurs lead to the same place. If you want to add some distance to your hike, turn left, as this is the longer way to follow the loop around and will add about 300 feet to your hike. Or if you're running or really want to add some distance, you can complete the full 0.2-mile circle. For a shorter hike, and the route featured here, stay to the right (north) and follow the east loop downhill 100 feet to another junction in the trail. This is where the other side of the loop meets up with the main trail. Stay straight (north) and continue on the east loop.

In the next 0.7 mile, the trail curves around to the left (northwest) and passes the Magnolia Cottage on the right. The east side of Lake Johnson comes back into view on the left side of the trail, shortly after passing Magnolia Cottage, and you reach a split in the trail. To the right, a spur trail crosses Lake Dam Road. Stay straight (north) and follow the trail around to the left and across the metal-railed arched bridge, which crosses over the east side of the lake. On the other side of the bridge, the trail follows along the top of a concrete berm and then veers to the left (west) before continuing behind a row of apartments and homes on the right. The trail continues for 0.9 mile along the north shore of Lake Johnson until you return to the trailhead.

Nearby Attractions

Six miles south is Hemlock Bluffs Nature Preserve (see page 66), with almost 4 miles of hiking trails. The trails in Hemlock Bluffs are similar in difficulty to the east loop of the Walnut Creek Trail. The trails at Hemlock traverse small hills and lead to steep bluffs with views of Swift Creek below. The park, designated to protect eastern hemlocks on the north-facing bluffs, features a nature center geared toward children.

Ten miles to the west of Lake Johnson Park is Fred G. Bond Metro Park (see pages 50 and 55), a 310-acre park with more than 4 miles of walking and biking trails that center on Bond Lake. The park is also the intersection for several of Cary's greenway trails, including the Black Creek Greenway, Oxford Hunt Greenway, and White Oak Greenway. Swift Creek Bluffs Nature Preserve (see page 111) is 2.6 miles southwest of Lake Johnson Park. The small 23-acre preserve has a 1.2-mile trail that follows along Swift Creek to the bluffs.

Directions

From the I-40/I-440 beltline, take Exit 295/Gorman Street. From Gorman Street, head south (away from North Carolina). Come to the intersection of Gorman Street and Tryon Road, and take a right onto Tryon Road. Go approximately 1 mile on Tryon and take a right onto Avent Ferry Road. Follow Avent Ferry Road 1.1 miles, crossing a bridge and going over the lake. Lake Johnson Park will be on the right, immediately after the bridge.

Raven Rock State Park:
Campbell Creek Loop Trail

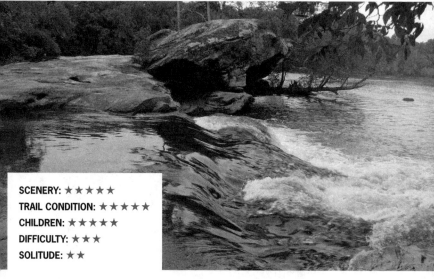

SCENERY: ★ ★ ★ ★ ★
TRAIL CONDITION: ★ ★ ★ ★ ★
CHILDREN: ★ ★ ★ ★ ★
DIFFICULTY: ★ ★
SOLITUDE: ★ ★

A SPUR TRAIL LEADS TO LANIER FALLS ON THE CAPE FEAR RIVER.

GPS TRAILHEAD COORDINATES: N35° 27.837' W78° 54.820'

DISTANCE & CONFIGURATION: 4.9-mile balloon

HIKING TIME: 2.5 hours

HIGHLIGHTS: Campbell Creek, Lanier Falls, and Cape Fear River

ELEVATION: 350' at trailhead to 138' at lowest point

ACCESS: Park: November–February: Daily, 8 a.m.–6 p.m. March–May and September–October: Daily, 8 a.m.–8 p.m. June–August: Daily, 8 a.m.–9 p.m. Closed December 25. Visitor center: Daily, 8 a.m.–5 p.m.; closed December 25. Free; campsites $13/day.

MAPS: Online at ncparks.gov or at the park's visitor center

FACILITIES: Restrooms, picnic areas, primitive campsites, auditorium, and classroom

WHEELCHAIR ACCESS: None

COMMENTS: This is a very popular trail with children and families. Avoid crowds by visiting the trail during weekdays. There are backcountry campsites along this trail. You can make it an overnight trip by reserving a site at the visitor center.

CONTACTS: 910-893-4888; ncparks.gov

Raven Rock State Park: Campbell Creek Loop Trail

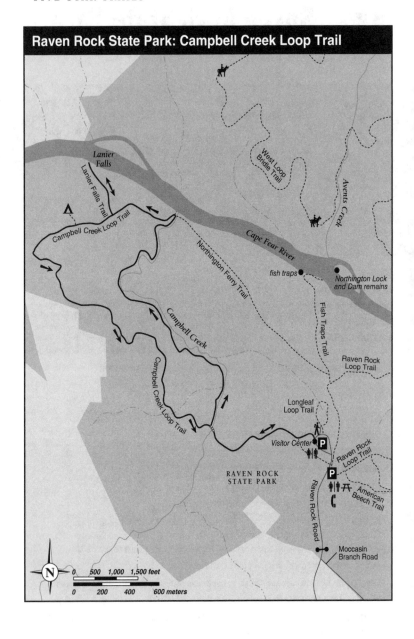

Lanier
Falls

West Loop
Bridle Trail

Avents Creek

Lanier Falls Trail

Campbell Creek Loop Trail

Cape Fear River

Northington Ferry Trail

fish traps

Northington Lock
and Dam remains

Campbell Creek

Fish Traps Trail

Raven Rock
Loop Trail

Campbell Creek Loop Trail

Longleaf
Loop Trail

Visitor Center

Raven Rock
Loop Trail

RAVEN ROCK
STATE PARK

American
Beech Trail

Raven Rock Road

Moccasin
Branch Road

N

0   500   1,000 1,500 feet

0   200   400   600 meters

Overview

This route follows the Campbell Creek Loop Trail and the Lanier Falls Trail to explore a large portion of the park's southwest section. The trail begins at the parking lot at the end of Raven Rock Road. You cross over Campbell Creek and then follow alongside the creek. Once you reach Cape Fear River, you have excellent views of the high bluffs that line the riverbank. A spur trail leads to Lanier Falls, a small fall near the bank of the Cape Fear River. Here a small rocky peninsula can be accessed on the other side of the falls. This bit of land that juts into the wide river is a popular fishing spot and a great place for a picnic, swimming, and sunning. Past the falls you reach another spur trail that leads to backcountry campsites, so you can turn your day hike into an overnight camping trip. This is a great route if you're looking for an introduction to backpacking or an overnight fishing or camping trip. The path explores a pine-and-oak forest before returning to the parking lot and visitor center.

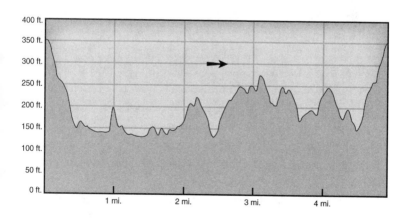

Route Details

Spring is a wonderful time to visit Raven Rock. While traversing the forest and floodplains along the riverbank, you can experience a variety of wildflowers, including Solomon's seal, Dutchman's-breeches, trailing arbutus, and spring beauties. You can also discover the exceptional diversity of landscapes within the park along this trail. At the trailhead and in the dry uplands, you hike through oak, pine, and hickory forests. As you approach the river you enter the floodplain, where you will encounter the largest trees along the path, mostly sycamores, beeches, and birches.

Along the steep riverbanks, water-loving rhododendrons, mountain laurels, elms, and maples take root. You can also search for elusive salamanders along these bluffs. In the streams you will find a wide variety of fish, turtles, beavers, muskrats, and other invertebrates. In the forests you are likely to encounter white-tailed deer, cottontails, fence lizards, hognose snakes, water snakes, and occasionally the venomous copperhead.

The trailhead to the Campbell Creek Loop Trail is a short walk from the visitor center and the main parking lot. Follow the small gravel path that starts on the far side of the parking lot, directly across from the visitor center. Follow the path for 150 feet until you reach a junction at the edge of the woods. This is the Campbell Creek Loop Trail. Turn right (northwest) onto the 4-foot-wide dirt path, which enters the forest and descends toward Campbell Creek. The trail is marked with blue circles on the trees. After 0.4 mile you reach a wooden boardwalk that crosses Campbell Creek. At the end of the boardwalk you reach a split in the trail. This is the beginning of the actual loop. Stay to the right (north) and follow the trail that narrows to a 2-foot-wide dirt path. Here the trail begins to follow alongside Campbell Creek, and you will find ferns growing along the trail's edge.

After 0.7 mile, the path leaves the edge of the creek. Over the next 0.4 mile, the trail climbs a small hill before rejoining the creek edge again. Continue an additional 0.2 mile until you reach a junction with a spur trail on your right, which leads down to Cape Fear River. Turn left (southwest) and follow the sign at this junction, continuing on the Campbell Creek Loop Trail toward Wilderness Camp. After 0.3 mile you will reach the junction with the short Lanier Falls Trail. Take the spur to the right (north) and follow the trail down to the edge of the Cape Fear River and Lanier Falls 0.2 mile away. After enjoying the area and the falls, turn around (south) and follow the spur trail for 0.2 mile back to the junction with the Campbell Creek Loop Trail. Turn right (west) and walk 0.2 mile until you reach the Wilderness Camp. A spur trail leads down to a string of private campsites nestled in the forest. The campsites are set off far enough from the spur trail to provide privacy and give the camper a fine wilderness experience, and the dense forest separating the campsites also contributes to the feeling of solitude.

If you are not camping, then continue straight on the Campbell Creek Loop Trail. After 0.2 mile the trail turns sharply to the left and begins heading south toward Campbell Creek. Continue through the pine-and-oak forest for 1.3 miles until you reach the junction that leads you back to the parking lot. Stay straight (west) and walk across the wooden boardwalk again. Follow the trail for 0.5 mile until you reach the parking lot and the visitor center where you started.

Nearby Attractions

The 174-acre Historic Yates Mill County Park (see page 82) is 36 miles northeast of Raven Rock State Park. The park has more than 2 miles of hiking trails, which circle around a 20-acre pond fed by Steep Hill Creek and its tributaries, that explore the park's surrounding wetlands and forests. The main feature of the park is Yates Mill, a masterfully restored 18th-century water-powered gristmill. Built by Samuel Pearson sometime between 1763 and 1778, the gristmill is the only fully operational water-powered gristmill in Wake County.

The 680-acre Harris Lake County Park (see page 60) is 38 miles north of Raven Rock State Park in New Hill, North Carolina. The park has more than 7 miles of hiking trails, more than 10 miles of mountain biking trails, a disc golf course, and boat ramps leading to the surrounding Harris Lake. Most of the hiking trails explore the shore of the lake peninsula and traverse longleaf-pine forests.

Directions

From Raleigh, take Capital Boulevard to US 401 South and follow it 16.6 miles. Turn left onto North Judd Parkway Northeast and follow it 2.1 miles. Turn left onto South Main Street/US 401 and follow it 11.9 miles. Turn right onto North Main Street/US 421 and follow it 1.6 miles. Turn right onto West Front Street/US 421 and follow it 6.2 miles. Turn right onto Raven Rock Road and follow it 3.1 miles. Raven Rock State Park will be on your left. If you reach the end of Raven Rock Road, you've gone too far.

From Durham, take NC 147 South and merge onto I-40 via Exit 5A toward RDU Airport/Raleigh; follow I-40 for 13.3 miles. Take Exit 293 toward Cary/Wake Forest, and then merge onto US 1 South via Exit 293A toward Cary/Asheboro; follow US 1 for 6.8 miles. Take the NC 55 East exit, Exit 95, toward Holly Springs/Fuquay-Varina. Turn left onto NC 55 East/East Williams Street and follow it 1.5 miles. NC 55 East/East Williams Street becomes NC 55 Bypass East; follow the bypass 4.7 miles. The bypass ends, but continue to follow NC 55 East for 3.8 miles. Turn right onto NC 55/North Ennis Street and follow it 0.1 mile. Take the first right onto North Main Street/US 401 and follow US 401 for 13.5 miles. Turn right onto North Main Street/US 421 South and follow it 1.6 miles. Turn right onto West Front Street/US 421 and follow US 421 for 6.2 miles. Turn right onto Raven Rock Road and follow it 3.1 miles. Raven Rock State Park will be on your left. If you reach the end of Raven Rock Road, you've gone too far.

14

Raven Rock State Park:
Raven Rock Loop

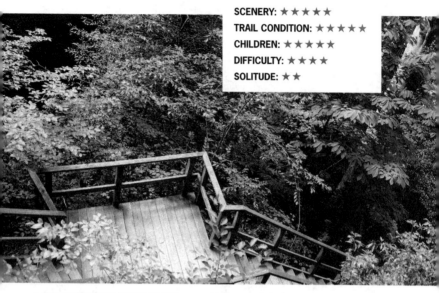

SCENERY: ★ ★ ★ ★ ★
TRAIL CONDITION: ★ ★ ★ ★ ★
CHILDREN: ★ ★ ★ ★ ★
DIFFICULTY: ★ ★ ★ ★
SOLITUDE: ★ ★

A BOARDWALK DESCENDS TO THE IMPRESSIVE RAVEN ROCK.

GPS TRAILHEAD COORDINATES: N35° 27.863' W78° 54.820'

DISTANCE & CONFIGURATION: 2.5-mile loop

HIKING TIME: 1.5 hours

HIGHLIGHTS: Cape Fear River, Raven Rock, and overlook

ELEVATION: 348' at trailhead to 123' at lowest point

ACCESS: Park: November–February: Daily, 8 a.m.–6 p.m. March–May and September–October: Daily, 8 a.m.–8 p.m. June–August: Daily, 8 a.m.–9 p.m. Closed December 25. Visitor center: Daily, 8 a.m.–5 p.m.; closed December 25. Free; campsites $13/day.

MAPS: Online at ncparks.gov or at the park's visitor center

FACILITIES: Restrooms, picnic areas, primitive campsites, auditorium, and classroom

WHEELCHAIR ACCESS: None

COMMENTS: This is a very popular trail with children and families. Avoid crowds by visiting on a weekday. The staircase leading down to Raven Rock can be quite strenuous on the way back up. Please take your limitations into account when considering this trail.

CONTACTS: 910-893-4888; ncparks.gov

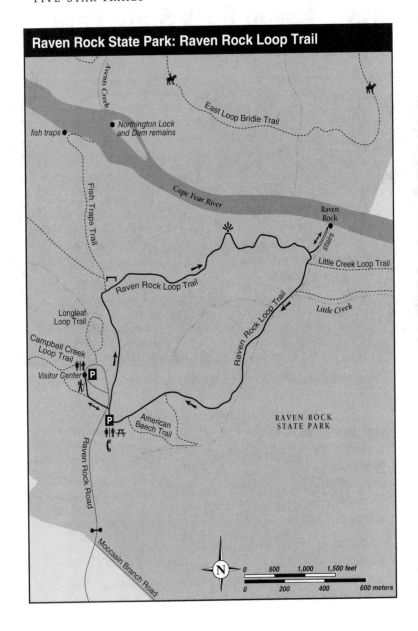

Raven Rock State Park: Raven Rock Loop Trail

Arents Creek

fish traps ●

● Northington Lock and Dam remains

East Loop Bridle Trail

Cape Fear River

Fish Traps Trail

Raven Rock

stairs

Little Creek Loop Trail

Raven Rock Loop Trail

Little Creek

Longleaf Loop Trail

Raven Rock Loop Trail

Campbell Creek Loop Trail

Visitor Center P

P

American Beech Trail

RAVEN ROCK STATE PARK

Raven Rock Road

Moccasin Branch Road

N

0   500   1,000   1,500 feet

0   200   400   600 meters

Overview

This route in the southeast section of the park follows the Raven Rock Loop Trail and leads to the namesake Raven Rock, an impressive crystalline rock formation that reaches up to 150 feet high and stretches more than a mile down the Cape Fear River. The trail begins at the parking lot at the end of Raven Rock Road and travels through oak, pine, and hickory upland forest. Closer to the Cape Fear River the trail winds through a floodplain forest of sycamore, beech, and birch trees. The path then arrives at an overlook that offers spectacular views of the steep rhododendron- and mountain laurel–covered bluffs that comprise the riverbanks below. The route follows the crest of these bluffs alongside the Cape Fear River and descends a series of wooden steps to the Raven Rock formation. Before circling back around to the parking lot, you can extend the hike by exploring the American Beech Trail through a large and impressive beech grove.

Route Details

The intriguing rock formations here were formed by the violent waters and swirling winds that have eroded this landscape over the

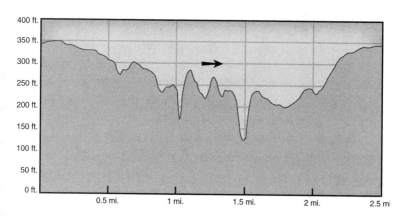

past 400 million years. Originally called Peterson's Rock after a settler who sought refuge among the overhanging ledges after his canoe overturned, the rock formation had its name officially changed in 1854 in honor of the flocks of ravens that used to roost here. Before Scottish settlers moved to this area, the surrounding lands were used for hunting grounds by the Siouan and Tuscarora American Indian tribes. Later the rock formations were used as a reliable landmark by riverboat captains who navigated the river with cargo. The locks and dams used in the river commerce enterprises can still be seen in the park today but were mostly destroyed by a hurricane in 1889. During the late 1880s, railroads were replacing river transports, and with river commerce becoming obsolete, the locks and dams were never repaired. From that point on the area that is now Raven Rock State Park was mainly used for recreation. Local residents organized and petitioned for the area to be preserved. In 1969 these community-led groups succeeded, and a bill was passed to designate this area as a state park. When the park was originally dedicated, it was only 390 acres. Today, through purchases and donations, the park has grown to 4,667 acres of preserved parkland.

The Raven Rock Loop Trailhead is a short walk from the visitor center and the main parking lot. From the visitor center, follow the gravel path that starts on the east side of the building. Follow the path for 0.1 mile around the edge of the parking lot until you reach a junction. To the left the gravel path continues alongside the road. Turn right—the trail will soon veer left, or southeast—and follow the trail for 300 feet until you reach a junction with a very wide dirt road. Turn left and follow the dirt road 60 feet to the Raven Rock Loop Trailhead.

The trail here becomes a 5-foot-wide dirt path and continues to the north through a mostly pine-and-oak forest. The trails in Raven Rock State Park are very well maintained, and the Raven Rock Loop Trail is well marked with red circular reflective disks posted on trees along the path. After 0.3 mile you reach a junction where the trail splits in two directions. There is a trash can here, as well as a bench for resting. Straight ahead, the trail becomes the Fish Traps Trail.

Veer right (east) toward Raven Rock. During this section the trail traverses several small hills. As the trail moves closer to the Cape Fear River, you will start to notice changes in the forest as it transitions from mostly pine to a denser and scrubbier oak composition that is commonly found in river-corridor forests in this area.

After 0.5 mile you will reach a very short spur trail on your left that leads downhill to an overlook. A wooden platform with handrails has been built atop the edge of the bluff and provides stunning views of the rocky bluffs that line the Cape Fear River below, which stretches off into the distance to the east and west. Follow the spur trail back to the Raven Rock Loop Trail and continue 0.3 mile until you reach the junction with the spur trail that leads down to Raven Rock. Turn left (northeast) on the spur trail toward Raven Rock. After 350 feet you reach the start of a long wooden staircase that leads down the steep hillside to the Cape Fear River and the base of Raven Rock. After walking down the 125-foot-long staircase, you reach the impressive Raven Rock. You can explore the bank of Cape Fear River and marvel at the Raven Rock towering above you before turning around and heading back up the steep stairs and back to the junction with the spur trail 500 feet away.

Once you reach the junction with the Raven Rock Loop Trail, stay straight (southwest) and head toward the parking lot. Continue on the Raven Rock Loop Trail for 250 feet until you reach the junction with the Little Creek Loop Trail. Stay straight and continue toward the parking lot and the Raven Rock Loop Trailhead. After walking just 370 feet, you will reach another junction with the Little Creek Loop Trail. Turn right (south) and continue on the wider gravel trail, passing an area with five picnic tables. Follow the path for 0.6 mile until you reach the junction with the American Beech Trail. If you want to extend the length of this trail, you can continue on the American Beech Trail, which traverses a large and impressive grove of beech trees. By continuing around the American Beech Trail, you will add an extra 0.5 mile to your hike. It's an easy and level hike, so why not? However, for the route described here, stay straight, and after an additional

0.1 mile on the Raven Rock Loop Trail, you reach a large picnic pavilion and restrooms on the right. Continue on the dirt path to the edge of the parking lot 0.1 mile away. From here you can return to the main parking lot and the visitor center by following the way you came in. Just follow the wide dirt path that runs north along the road toward the visitor center. This will lead you back to the gravel path. The visitor center and the main parking lot will be straight ahead.

Nearby Attractions

The 174-acre Historic Yates Mill County Park (see page 82) is 36 miles northeast of Raven Rock State Park. The park has more than 2 miles of hiking trails that circle a 20-acre pond fed by Steep Hill Creek and its tributaries, exploring the park's surrounding wetlands and forests. The main feature of the park is Yates Mill, a masterfully restored 18th-century water-powered gristmill. Built by Samuel Pearson sometime between 1763 and 1778, the gristmill is the only fully operational water-powered gristmill in Wake County.

The 680-acre Harris Lake County Park (see page 60) is 38 miles north of Raven Rock State Park in New Hill, North Carolina. The park has more than 7 miles of hiking trails, more than 10 miles of mountain-biking trails, a disc golf course, and boat ramps leading to the surrounding Harris Lake. Most of the hiking trails explore the shore of the lake peninsula and traverse longleaf-pine forests.

Directions

From Raleigh, take Capital Boulevard to US 401 South and follow it 16.6 miles. Turn left onto North Judd Parkway Northeast and follow it 2.1 miles. Turn left onto South Main Street/US 401and follow it 11.9 miles. Turn right onto North Main Street/US 421 and follow it 1.6 miles. Turn right onto West Front Street/US 421 and follow it 6.2 miles. Turn right onto Raven Rock Road and follow it 3.1 miles. Raven Rock State Park will be on your left. If you reach the end of Raven Rock Road, you've gone too far.

From Durham, take NC 147 South and merge onto I-40 via Exit 5A toward RDU Airport/Raleigh; follow I-40 for 13.3 miles. Take Exit 293 toward Cary/Wake Forest, and then merge onto US 1 South via Exit 293A toward Cary/Asheboro; follow US 1 for 6.8 miles. Take the NC 55 East exit, Exit 95, toward Holly Springs/Fuquay-Varina. Turn left onto NC 55 East/East Williams Street and follow it 1.5 miles. NC 55 East/East Williams Street becomes NC 55 Bypass East; follow the bypass 4.7 miles. The bypass ends, but continue to follow NC 55 East for 3.8 miles. Turn right onto NC 55/North Ennis Street and follow it 0.1 mile. Take the first right onto North Main Street/US 401 and follow US 401 for 13.5 miles. Turn right onto North Main Street/US 421 South and follow it 1.6 miles. Turn right onto West Front Street/US 421 and follow US 421 for 6.2 miles. Turn right onto Raven Rock Road and follow it 3.1 miles. Raven Rock State Park will be on your left. If you reach the end of Raven Rock Road, you've gone too far.

15

Shelley Lake:
Sertoma Park

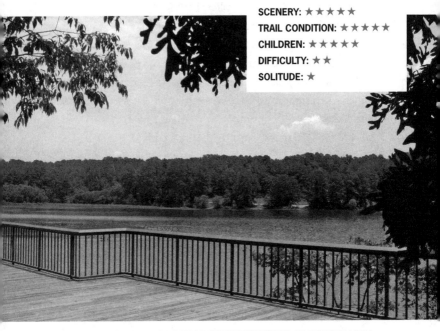

SCENERY: ★ ★ ★ ★
TRAIL CONDITION: ★ ★ ★ ★ ★
CHILDREN: ★ ★ ★ ★ ★
DIFFICULTY: ★ ★
SOLITUDE: ★

AN OBSERVATION DECK OFFERS PICTURESQUE VIEWS OF SHELLEY LAKE.

GPS TRAILHEAD COORDINATES: N35° 43.234' W78° 41.262'

DISTANCE & CONFIGURATION: 1.3-mile loop

HIKING TIME: 1 hour

HIGHLIGHTS: Shelley Lake and art center

ELEVATION: 317' at trailhead to 250' at lowest point

ACCESS: Daily, sunrise–sunset; free

MAPS: Online at raleighnc.gov and at the park visitor center

FACILITIES: Restrooms, picnic pavilions, water fountains, playground, sports fields, exercise stations, art center, and boathouse

WHEELCHAIR ACCESS: Yes

COMMENTS: This trail is shared with bikers, runners, and walkers and is very popular with families and children. To avoid crowds, visit the park in the early morning on weekdays.

CONTACTS: 919-420-2331; raleighnc.gov

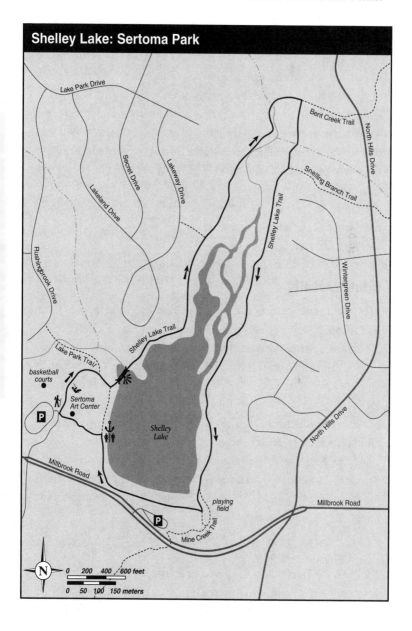

Shelley Lake: Sertoma Park

Lake Park Drive

Bent Creek Trail

North Hills Drive

Secret Drive

Lakeway Drive

Lakeland Drive

Snelling Branch Trail

Shelley Lake Trail

Wintergreen Drive

Rushingbrook Drive

Lake Park Trail

Shelley Lake Trail

basketball
courts

Sertoma
Art Center

P

North Hills Drive

*Shelley
Lake*

Millbrook Road

Millbrook Road

playing
field

P

Mine Creek Trail

N

0   200   400   600 feet

0   50   100   150 meters

Overview

Just 6 miles north of downtown Raleigh and just outside the suburb of Brookhaven, the 53-acre Shelley Lake Park has more than 2 miles of paved trails that circle the forested lakeshore, making it an excellent escape from the city for a quick run or leisurely walk in a serene setting. This route starts to the east of the lake at Optimist Park and follows the paved Snelling Branch Trail through a forested corridor to the Shelley Lake Trail. You circle Shelley Lake through quiet woods, with exceptional views of the lake and plenty of opportunities to encounter the resident waterfowl and wildlife. Along the way you'll pass workout stations, a playground area, three sports fields, and the Sertoma Art Center.

Route Details

Many spur trails connect to the Shelley Lake Trail, and most of them lead into nearby neighborhoods. To extend the trail to a more than 3-mile round-trip, you can start from the parking lot for the Bent Creek Trail to the north of the lake, at the Snelling Branch Trail at Optimist Park to the east of the lake, or at the Ironwood Trail parking lot to the south of the lake. While visiting the park, you can also rent boats and paddle around the lake. The park offers loaner fishing poles and tackle for free, and the boathouse sells tackle and bait.

The Sertoma Art Center offers classes for adults and kids in painting, drawing, fiber arts, and pottery. The center has an outstanding complete black-and-white darkroom studio for photographers and offers classes in music, dance, and fitness.

This route starts from the trailhead on the east side of the parking lot in front of the Sertoma Art Center. From the trailhead for the Shelley Lake Trail, follow the paved spur trail past the playground on your right for 0.1 mile until you reach the junction with the Lake Park Trail, a 0.4-mile unpaved trail that runs to the north. Stay straight and descend to the lake for 220 feet until you reach the Shelley Lake Trail at the lakeshore. Turn left (northeast) and start on the Shelley Lake

Trail. You immediately come to a long bridge that crosses a small arm of the lake. This is a favorite spot for fishing and taking in the views of the lake that stretch to the north and south. A large observation deck on the left side of the trail protrudes from the bridge. Continue on the Shelley Lake Trail, following the edge of the lakeshore for 0.4 mile, until you reach a junction with a spur trail that leads to Lakeway Drive. Stay straight (northeast) and continue on Shelley Lake Trail. After 0.1 mile the trail reaches the edge of the creek and follows alongside the creek for 0.2 mile, where you reach the junction with the Bent Creek Trail. Turn right (south), heading back toward the main body of Shelley Lake. Follow the east side of the creek for 0.1 mile until you arrive at another junction with a spur trail that leads into the neighborhood to the east of the trail. Stay straight on the Shelley Lake Trail. The trail follows along the east side of the creek, and after 0.3 mile you reach the lakeshore again. Continue for 0.3 mile, passing a sports field on the left, until you reach a junction with a spur trail that leads across Millbrook Road to a parking lot and the southern trailhead of the Shelley Lake Trail. Stay straight (south) on the Shelley Lake Trail. After 60 feet the Shelley Lake Trail takes a sharp turn to the right (west) and goes over a man-made berm at the edge of the lake. After 0.2 mile the trail turns sharply to the right (north), still following along the lakeshore. Walk 450 feet until you reach the Sertoma Art Center. Turn left (west) and follow the wooden steps up to the art center and the parking lot where you started your hike.

Nearby Attractions

Six miles west of Shelley Lake is William B. Umstead State Park (see pages 117 and 123). This 5,579-acre park offers more than 20 miles of hiking trails, as well as opportunities for paddling and boating on Big Lake, and biking and horseback riding on the bridle and biking trails throughout the park. Umstead also has tent and trailer camping for $20 per day. Showers, water, and restrooms are located in the campgrounds.

Falls Lake State Recreation Area, with a 12,000-acre lake and 26,000 acres of woodlands, offers more than 20 miles of hiking trails, including a portion of the Mountains-to-Sea Trail that traverses the south shore of the lake, as well as other shorter trails at Beaver Dam, B. W. Wells, Holly Point, Rolling View, and Sandling Beach. The 1-mile loop trail at B. W. Wells passes the naturalist's home (see page 163). The entrance to Falls Lake State Recreation Area is 12 miles north of Shelley Lake.

Blue Jay Point County Park (see page 26), a 236-acre park located on the shores of Falls Lake in northern Wake County, offers more than 5 miles of trails within its boundaries, as well as open play fields, playgrounds, an environmental education center, and an overnight lodge. The park features hiking trails that also connect with the Falls Lake State Recreation Area trails to offer longer hiking opportunities. The park is 10 miles north of Shelley Lake Park.

Directions

From Raleigh, the park is 6 miles north of downtown. Take the Glenwood Avenue North/US 70 West ramp and merge onto Glenwood Avenue/US 70 East. Follow US 70 East for 3.4 miles. Turn right onto Lead Mine Road and follow it 1.3 miles. Turn right onto West Millbrook Road and follow it 0.6 mile. The entrance to Shelley Lake Park will be on your left. If you reach Oldtowne Road, you've gone too far.

From Durham, the park is 18 miles southeast of downtown. From Holloway Street take US 70 East toward Raleigh and follow it 11.8 miles. Turn left onto West Millbrook Road and follow it 3.1 miles. The entrance to Shelley Lake Park will be on your left. If you reach Oldtowne Road, you've gone too far.

16 # Swift Creek Bluffs
Nature Preserve

SCENERY: ★ ★ ★ ★
TRAIL CONDITION: ★ ★ ★ ★ ★
CHILDREN: ★ ★ ★
DIFFICULTY: ★ ★
SOLITUDE: ★ ★ ★ ★

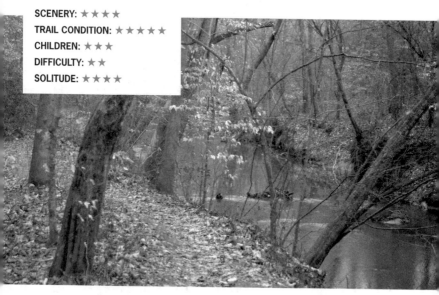

JOURNEY THROUGH AN OVERCUP OAK SWAMP AND ALONG SWIFT CREEK.

GPS TRAILHEAD COORDINATES: N35° 43.058' W78° 45.195'

DISTANCE & CONFIGURATION: 0.9-mile balloon

HIKING TIME: 1 hour

HIGHLIGHTS: Swift Creek, old-growth beech forest, bluffs, and plant diversity

ELEVATION: Negligible—302' at trailhead to 297' at lowest point

ACCESS: 24/7 but recommended only during daylight hours; free

MAPS: At triangleland.org and at the trailhead kiosk

FACILITIES: None

WHEELCHAIR ACCESS: None

COMMENTS: The parking lot to the preserve is easy to miss even though it sits right off the road. Keep an eye out for the wastewater station that is right next to the parking lot, and remember that the parking lot is just on the other side of Swift Creek Bridge. The preserve sees few visitors during the week and is fairly isolated, so while it's a nice place to take a quiet walk, take extra precautions if you're hiking alone.

CONTACTS: 919-833-3662; triangleland.org

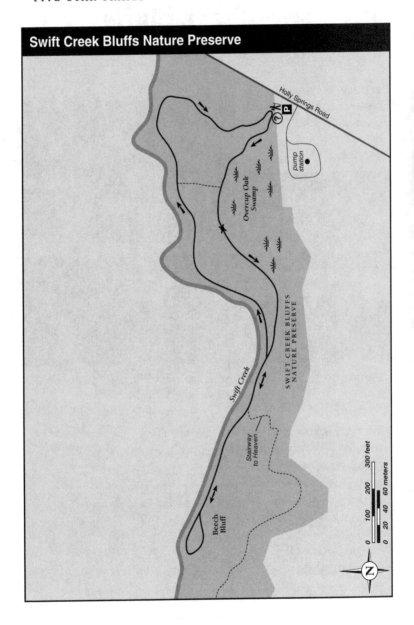

Swift Creek Bluffs Nature Preserve

Overview

Swift Creek Bluffs Nature Preserve is a 23-acre park 5 miles south of downtown Cary. The nature preserve is protected by the Triangle Land Conservancy, which has done a remarkable job of protecting more than 10,000 acres of land in the Triangle area. This hike is nearly 1 mile and takes you through all of the preserve's distinct habitats. A floodplain makes up most of the basin of the preserve, and when the rainfall is exceptionally high, water often flows over the steeply cut riverbank and floods the low-lying land that surrounds Swift Creek. In this bottomland you will find a hardwood forest of swamp chestnut oaks, bitternut hickories, and American elms. On the slopes of the surrounding bluffs that rise beside the trail, you will find a collection of old-growth beech trees that have survived the selective timber harvesting that occurred in this area over the last 100 years. The trail leaves the parking lot and quickly reaches the base of the bluffs. The path then follows along the bank of Swift Creek and beside the towering bluffs to a clearing that overlooks the creek. On the return hike the trail loops through a flat, low-lying floodplain and beech grove before returning to the trailhead and parking lot.

Route Details

Park your vehicle at the small lot in front of the trailhead kiosk. If the lot is full, park along the road. The trail starts to the left (west) of the kiosk, where the trail crosses a small footbridge. The dirt path is about 4 feet wide and enters into the forest. Follow the path for 200 feet until you come to a junction in the trail. To the right (north) the trail loops through a bottomland beech flat. Stay straight (west) and follow the trail for 150 feet, passing the low-lying swamp filled with overcup oaks on the left, until you reach another split in the trail.

The area now known as Swift Creek Bluffs Nature Preserve was discovered nearly by accident. A botany student from nearby North Carolina State University was walking his dog along the creek and took notice of the exceptional diversity of habitats that occupied this relatively small area of land surrounding Swift Creek. The student informed botany professors at the university about the living museum he had stumbled upon and also noted the existence of an old-growth forest on the slopes of the bluffs. Several years later, the Triangle Land Conservancy recognized the uniqueness of the Swift Creek Basin and the value in protecting this particular area of land.

At the trail junction, the trail reaches Swift Creek. Off to the left you can see the base of the bluff system start to appear and rise beside Swift Creek's bank. To the right (northeast), the trail loops back around through the flat floodplain and returns to the trailhead and parking lot. If you want to shorten the trail at this point, you can turn right and follow the loop back to the trailhead. For a longer hike, stay straight (west) and cross the small wooden footbridge.

Over the next 0.3 mile the trail follows the bank of Swift Creek, and the bluffs rise higher and higher to the left side of trail. The trail crosses a 20-foot-long wooden footbridge. At the beginning of the bridge, you will find a metal plaque with the poem "Wild Peace" inscribed on it; in my opinion, the poem is definitely worth reading. After crossing the bridge, the trail gently climbs to the bank of Swift Creek. Continue for 0.2 mile until you reach another split in the trail. If you veer left (west), the trail climbs a very steep hill via a long set of wooden steps; these steps are called the Stairway to Heaven and lead to the edge of the preserve, where the trail connects with the Birkhaven Greenway Trail. Instead, veer to the right (northwest) and continue alongside Swift Creek for 0.1 mile until you reach the large clearing on the bank of the creek.

This clearing, elevated above the creek, offers great views of the side of the bluffs and Swift Creek below. It is a great spot for a picnic or just to stop and relax for a while in the heart of the preserve. After enjoying the view, you can turn around and head back (southeast) the way you came in and continue toward the trailhead, following alongside Swift Creek. After 0.1 mile the trail splits. If you stay straight, you continue back to the trailhead. However, veer to the left (northeast) and follow alongside Swift Creek. This section of the trail traverses a low-lying forested floodplain, dotted with beech trees. This type of habitat is known as a beech flat. In springtime this area of the preserve is especially colorful. The rich nutrients that are deposited when the creek overflows provide the sustaining elements for a medley of wildflowers that grow in the floodplain. Here you will find trout lilies, mayapples, jack-in-the-pulpits, atamasco lilies, and the aptly named spring beauties.

After 0.2 mile you reach another split in the trail. If you want to make the trail shorter, you can turn right (south) and take a shortcut to the parking lot and trailhead by following this trail through the middle of the preserve. To continue on the longer hike, however, stay straight (east) and continue following the loop through the beech flat for 0.1 mile until you reach the trailhead and parking lot.

Nearby Attractions

Three miles north of Swift Creek Bluffs Nature Preserve, you can take the North Harrison Avenue exit off of I-40 and visit the William B. Umstead State Park (see pages 117 and 123). This 5,579-acre park offers more than 20 miles of hiking trails, as well as opportunities for paddling and boating on Big Lake, and biking and horseback riding on the bridle and biking trails throughout the park. Umstead also has tent and trailer camping for $20 per day. Showers, water, and restrooms are located in the campgrounds.

Four miles to the southwest of Swift Creek Bluffs Nature Preserve is Hemlock Bluffs Nature Preserve (see page 66), which offers nearly 3 miles of hiking trails through a very well-maintained and beautiful park and was established to protect rare eastern hemlock trees on the north-facing bluffs. The park has an impressive 3,700-square-foot nature center that offers various programs geared toward children, as well as restrooms, water fountains, a gift shop, and a lecture hall.

Directions

From I-40, take Exit 293A, a 0.5-mile multiexit ramp toward Sanford, US 1 South, and US 64 West. Take the second exit, Exit 101A/Walnut Street/Shopping Centers, off of the extended ramp. Turn right on Walnut Street, passing through the Crossroads shopping area. Follow Walnut Street 1.2 miles until you reach Tryon Road at a traffic signal. Go straight and continue following Walnut Street for 2.3 miles, passing the Swift Creek Bridge, and immediately find Swift Creek Bluffs Nature Preserve on the right. The preserve is adjacent to a Town of Cary lift station, and you can park in the gravel lot in front of the kiosk and trailhead.

17

William B. Umstead State Park: Oak Rock and Pott's Branch Trails

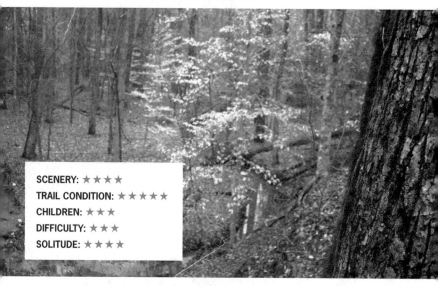

SCENERY: ★ ★ ★ ★
TRAIL CONDITION: ★ ★ ★ ★ ★
CHILDREN: ★ ★ ★
DIFFICULTY: ★ ★ ★
SOLITUDE: ★ ★ ★ ★

A LAUREL TREE BLOSSOMS BESIDE POTT'S BRANCH.

GPS TRAILHEAD COORDINATES: N35° 52.463' W78° 45.642'

DISTANCE & CONFIGURATION: 1.73-mile loop

HIKING TIME: 1.5 hours

HIGHLIGHTS: Pott's Branch, plant diversity, and wildflowers in spring and fall

ELEVATION: 400' at trailhead to 328' at lowest point

ACCESS: November–February: Daily, 8 a.m.–6 p.m. March–April and September–October: Daily, 8 a.m.–8 p.m. May–August: Daily, 8 a.m.–9 p.m. Closed December 25. Free.

MAPS: Online at ncparks.gov, at the Crabtree Creek entrance park office, and at the trailhead kiosk

FACILITIES: Restrooms, park office, playing field, campground, and boat rental

WHEELCHAIR ACCESS: None

COMMENTS: While bikers are allowed to ride on certain trails in the park, only foot traffic is allowed on this trail. Swimming in the lake is prohibited. Dogs are welcome in the park as long as they are kept on a leash no longer than 6 feet.

CONTACTS: 919-571-4170; ncparks.gov

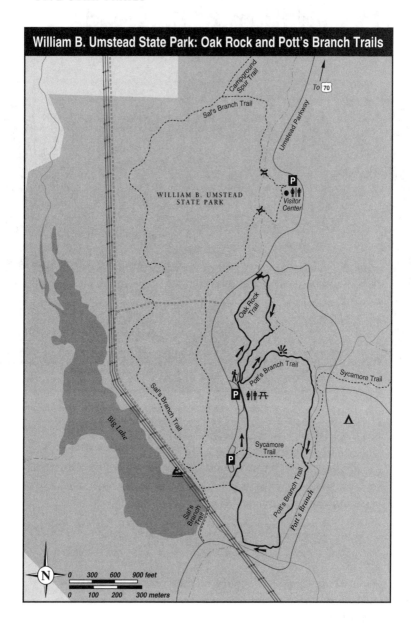

William B. Umstead State Park: Oak Rock and Pott's Branch Trails

Overview

William B. Umstead State Park is tightly nestled among the cities of Raleigh, Cary, Durham, and the Research Triangle Park. The park is divided into two sections: Crabtree Creek in the north and Reedy Creek in the south. This route combines two popular trails in the park, the Oak Rock Trail and the Pott's Branch Trail, to make an enjoyable loop that follows along the Pott's Branch stream and provides access to a spur trail that leads down to Big Lake. The route starts at the Oak Rock Trail, which loops around through a beautiful forest. It then connects with the Pott's Branch Trail, which descends to Pott's Branch and follows alongside the winding creek, eventually reaching the southern edge of Big Lake. From here the trail turns to the north and leads away from the lake, returning to the trailhead.

Route Details

Drive into the state park, pass the visitor center, and park your vehicle at the first lot on the left side of the road. The Oak Rock Trailhead is in the northeast corner of the lot and is marked by an orange sign. Two dirt paths lead into the forest. Stay straight (northeast) on the Oak Rock Trail, blazed with white squares. Interpretive plaques mark and describe several of the tree species found along the trail during this next section. To the left you can see the road, and to the right you can see the other side of the loop through the trees.

Follow the gently sloping trail for 0.3 mile to the stone bridge. Here the creek bends and winds through the forest. Cross the stone bridge and follow the trail alongside the creek. Continue for 0.2 mile until you reach a spur trail. The 35-foot spur trail leads to an interesting rock formation, surrounded by oak trees. After checking out the spur trail, continue to the left (southwest) on the Oak Rock Trail. The trail is well marked and very easy to follow. Continue on the loop trail for 0.2 mile until you come back to the Oak Rock Trailhead and parking lot where you began.

From here, follow the Pott's Branch Trail, marked with orange diamonds, uphill to the left (east). Continue uphill and around to the left until you reach a trail junction. Stay straight (east) on the Pott's Branch Trail toward the picnic area. The trail gently descends for 350 feet to a split in the trail. Stay to the left (east) and continue for 300 feet to the large observation deck.

During the 19th century, this forest was extensively cleared of trees and turned into farming fields. At first the farmers were successful, but after years of poor farming practices and a repetitive devotion to one-crop production, the soil was exhausted and no longer good for farming. During the Depression, farmers still tried to grow cotton in the worn-out soil around Crabtree Creek without much luck, and eventually the Civilian Conservation Corps, as well as the Works Progress Administration, helped construct four camps as well as day-use and picnic facilities in the park, which opened to the public in 1937.

The forest here is slowly being restored to its former greatness. In the park you may find deer, beavers, ducks, and raccoons. Along the park's streams, you will find rhododendrons and laurels, plants typically found in the mountains, and in every season there are a variety of trees, shrubs, ferns, and wildflowers in the surrounding forest.

After passing the observation deck with a view of the surrounding forest and the winding stream below, turn left (east) and follow the Pott's Branch Trail down the steep hill, keeping the observation deck to your left. While hiking downhill you pass a stream, Pott's Branch, on your left, winding through the forest. The trail descends to the stream and follows alongside Pott's Branch, passing on the left a small stone wall that once dammed the creek.

There are plenty of spots to sit beside the stream on this next section of trail, and they make a great place for resting or enjoying a picnic on a nice day. After 0.3 mile you reach the junction with the Sycamore Trail. Stay straight (south), heading uphill on the Pott's Branch Trail. This next 0.4-mile section traverses some small hills before the trail descends to a creek to the left of the trail. From here you climb uphill to the junction with a spur trail that leads to the Sal's Branch Trail. Stay to the right (northeast) and follow the Pott's Branch Trail up a small hill.

After 350 feet you reach a trail junction with the spur trail that leads to the southernmost parking lot along Umstead Parkway, the park's main entrance road. Turn right (north) toward the northern parking lot where you started. The path becomes paved and runs alongside the road. After 500 feet you reach a trail junction. Turn left (north) and continue on the paved path, passing the restrooms on the right, and return to the parking lot.

Nearby Attractions

William B. Umstead State Park (also see page 123) covers 5,579 acres and offers more than 20 miles of hiking trails, as well as opportunities for paddling and boating on Big Lake, and biking and horseback riding on the bridle and biking trails throughout the park. Umstead State Park also has tent and trailer camping for $20 per day. A campground is just past the Crabtree Creek entrance on the right side. Showers, water, and restrooms are located in the campground.

Seventeen miles to the south of William B. Umstead State Park is Hemlock Bluffs Nature Preserve (see page 66), which features nearly 3 miles of hiking trails through a very well-maintained and beautiful park. The preserve was established to protect rare eastern hemlock trees on the north-facing bluffs. The park has an impressive 3,700-square-foot nature center that offers various programs geared toward children, as well as restrooms, water fountains, a gift shop, and lecture hall.

Thirteen miles to the south of William B. Umstead State Park is Fred G. Bond Metro Park (see pages 50 and 55), a 310-acre park with more than 4 miles of walking and biking trails that center on Bond Lake. The park is also the intersection for several of Cary's greenway trails, including Black Creek Greenway, Oxford Hunt

Greenway, and White Oak Greenway. Swift Creek Bluffs Nature Preserve (see page 111) is 16 miles to the south of William B. Umstead State Park. The 23-acre preserve has a 1.2-mile trail that follows along Swift Creek to the bluffs.

Directions

William B. Umstead State Park is in Wake County, between Raleigh and Durham. The Crabtree Creek section is 10 miles northwest of Raleigh, off US 70. The park visitor center and camping facilities are in this section. From Raleigh, start out going northeast on Capital Boulevard and follow it 3.3 miles. Merge onto I-440 West toward Sanford and follow it 4.1 miles. Merge onto Glenwood Avenue/US 70 West via Exit 7B toward Crabtree Valley, and follow it 6.2 miles. Umstead Parkway and the entrance to William B. Umstead State Park, which leads to the park office and visitor center, will be on your left. If you reach Marvino Lane, you've gone about 0.1 mile too far. Follow Umstead Parkway 1.6 miles until you reach the Oak Rock Trailhead and parking lot, on the left side.

William B. Umstead
State Park: Sal's Branch Trail

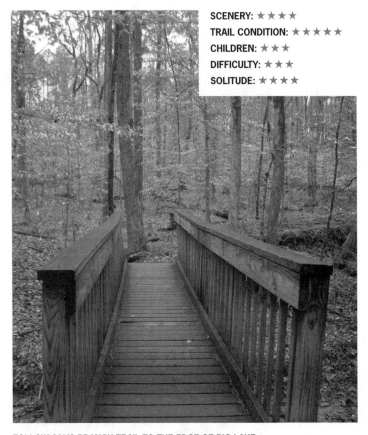

SCENERY: ★ ★ ★ ★
TRAIL CONDITION: ★ ★ ★ ★ ★
CHILDREN: ★ ★ ★
DIFFICULTY: ★ ★ ★
SOLITUDE: ★ ★ ★ ★

FOLLOW SAL'S BRANCH TRAIL TO THE EDGE OF BIG LAKE.

GPS TRAILHEAD COORDINATES: N35° 52.851' W78° 45.520'

DISTANCE & CONFIGURATION: 2.4-mile loop

HIKING TIME: 2 hours

HIGHLIGHTS: Big Lake

ELEVATION: 391' at trailhead to 437' at peak and 357' at lowest point

ACCESS: November–February: Daily, 8 a.m.–6 p.m. March–April and September–October:
Daily, 8 a.m.–8 p.m. May–August: Daily, 8 a.m.–9 p.m. Closed December 25. Free.

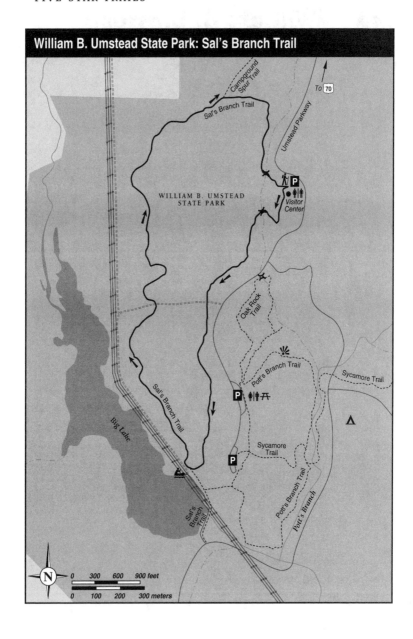

William B. Umstead State Park: Sal's Branch Trail

Campground Spur Trail

Sal's Branch Trail

To 70

Umstead Parkway

P

Visitor Center

WILLIAM B. UMSTEAD STATE PARK

Oak Rock Trail

Pott's Branch Trail

Sycamore Trail

Sal's Branch Trail

Big Lake

P

Sycamore Trail

P

Pott's Branch Trail

Pott's Branch

Sal's Branch Trail

N

| 0 | 300 | 600 | 900 feet |
| 0 | 100 | 200 | 300 meters |

MAPS: Online at ncparks.gov, at the Crabtree Creek entrance park office, and at the trailhead kiosk

FACILITIES: Restrooms, park office, playing field, campground, and boat rental

WHEELCHAIR ACCESS: None

COMMENTS: While bikers may ride on certain trails in the park, only foot traffic is allowed on this trail. Swimming in the lake is prohibited. Dogs are welcome in the park as long as they are kept on a leash no longer than 6 feet.

CONTACTS: 919-571-4170; ncparks.gov

Overview

William B. Umstead State Park is a forested oasis tightly nestled among the urban cities of Raleigh, Cary, Durham, and the Research Triangle Park. The park is divided into two sections: Crabtree Creek in the north and Reedy Creek in the south. This trail starts at the visitor-center parking lot, in the Crabtree Creek section of the park. You follow a spur trail to the Sal's Branch Trail and traverse a few small hills before reaching the southern edge of Big Lake. From here the trail follows the eastern shore of the lake, offering nice views of the lake to the left. Keeping the lake to your left and continuing straight on Sal's Branch Trail, you climb over a steep hill and then descend to the visitor center, where you started.

Route Details

Enter the park from the Crabtree Creek entrance, and park at the visitor-center lot (the first lot on the right after you enter the park). A spur trail leads from the kiosk in the northwest corner of the parking lot to the Sal's Branch Trailhead. The trail is blazed with orange circles, and a brown sign marks the trailhead well. Follow the trail downhill and immediately reach a trail junction. Turn left (south) and follow the trail behind the visitor center.

American bison, elk, bobcats, and wolves once inhabited this area. When Europeans began traveling through the area in the 18th century, Native Americans developed avenues of trade that included the Occoneechee Trail to the north and the Pee Dee Trail to the south. The first major move toward European settlement came in 1774, when land grants of large tracts of forested property were assigned to encourage agricultural growth and production. Once these early farmers exhausted the soil with poor farming techniques, federal and state agencies united to buy 5,000 acres of this submarginal land. In 1934 the agencies developed the Crabtree Creek Recreation Area, now known as William B. Umstead State Park.

In 1950 the park was separated into two different sections, with Crabtree Creek in the north and Reedy Creek—more than 1,000 acres established as a segregated park for African Americans—in the south. In 1966, the Crabtree Creek and Reedy Creek areas were combined under the single entity of William B. Umstead State Park, in honor of the conservation-minded Governor William Bradley Umstead, who fought hard to preserve the land and set it aside as a park for all to enjoy.

After 400 feet you reach the gravel overflow parking lot for the visitor center and Crabtree Creek trails. Follow the sign to the right (northwest) and walk across the parking lot to the 4-foot-wide unpaved path that leads into the forest. After crossing a small creek via a footbridge, you begin climbing uphill, the trail widening as you ascend. After 0.3 mile you reach a junction with a park service road. Stay straight (south) on the Sal's Branch Trail. During this next 0.4-mile section of the trail, you encounter several spur trails, but stay straight on Sal's Branch Trail. You also climb several small hills that offer nice views of the rolling forested landscape. Continue until you reach a gravel road and the edge of Big Lake. Turn right (northwest) and walk uphill, following the gravel road toward the power lines and following alongside the shore of Big Lake to your left.

Continue for 0.4 mile until you reach a junction with a park service road. Stay straight (north) and continue on the unpaved Sal's Branch Trail, which continues ascending gradually. Over the next 0.3 mile you climb to the highest elevation that you will reach on the trail: 437 feet. Once you reach the top of the hill, you can relax and breathe a bit easier, because from here you start a gradual descent all the way to the parking lot where you started.

From the top of the hill, continue another 0.3 mile down to the trail junction with the Campground Spur Trail. To the left (northeast) the Campground Spur Trail is an easy 0.4-mile walk to the Crabtree Creek Campground. Stay straight (southeast), though, to follow the Sal's Branch Trail as it curves to the right and reaches the bank of a small stream. Follow the trail, continuing 0.3 mile and crossing the creek over a pair of wooden bridges. Soon the trail curves around to the left (southeast) and reaches the gravel overflow parking lot again. Cross the parking lot and backtrack on the spur trail for 300 feet to return to the trailhead and your vehicle.

Nearby Attractions

William B. Umstead State Park (see also page 117) is 5,579 acres and offers more than 20 miles of hiking trails, as well as opportunities for paddling and boating on Big Lake, and biking and horseback riding on the bridle and biking trails throughout the park. Umstead State Park also has tent and trailer camping for $20 per day. A campground is just past the Crabtree Creek entrance on the right side. Showers, water, and restrooms are located in the campground.

Seventeen miles to the south of William B. Umstead State Park is Hemlock Bluffs Nature Preserve (see page 66), which offers nearly 3 miles of hiking trails through a very well-maintained and beautiful park. The preserve was established to protect rare eastern hemlock trees on the north-facing bluffs. The park has an impressive 3,700-square-foot nature center that offers various programs geared toward children, as well as restrooms, water fountains, a gift shop, and a lecture hall.

Thirteen miles to the south of William B. Umstead State Park is Fred G. Bond Metro Park (see pages 50 and 55), a 310-acre park with more than 4 miles of walking and biking trails that center on Bond Lake. The park is also the intersection for several of Cary's greenway trails, including Black Creek Greenway, Oxford Hunt Greenway, and White Oak Greenway. Swift Creek Bluffs Nature Preserve (see page 111) is 16 miles to the south of William B. Umstead State Park. The 23-acre preserve has a 1.2-mile trail that follows Swift Creek to the bluffs.

Directions

William B. Umstead State Park is in Wake County, between Raleigh and Durham. The Crabtree Creek section is 10 miles northwest of Raleigh, off US 70. The park visitor center and camping facilities are in this section. From Raleigh, start out going northeast on Capital Boulevard and follow it 3.3 miles. Merge onto I-440 West toward Sanford and follow it 4.1 miles. Merge onto Glenwood Avenue/US 70 West via Exit 7B toward Crabtree Valley, and follow it 6.2 miles. Umstead Parkway and the entrance to William B. Umstead State Park, which leads to the park office and visitor center, will be on your left. If you reach Marvino Lane, you've gone about 0.1 mile too far. Follow Umstead Parkway 1.6 miles until you reach the Sal's Branch Trailhead and parking lot, on the left side.

THE VISITOR CENTER AT WILLIAM B. UMSTEAD STATE PARK

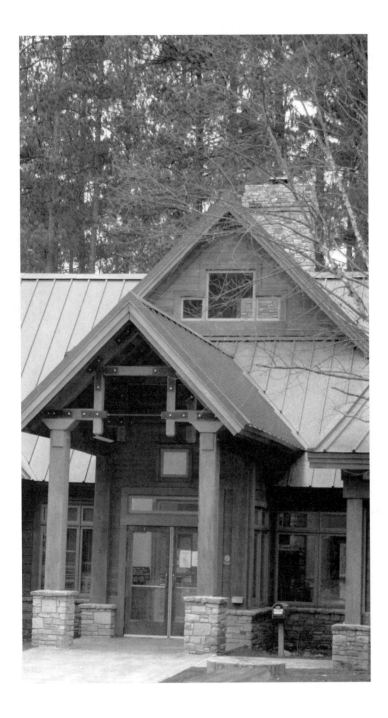

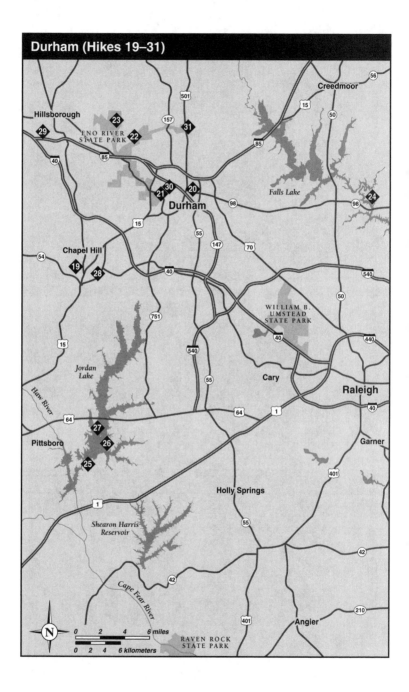

Durham (Hikes 19–31)

Creedmoor

Hillsborough

ENO RIVER STATE PARK

29

23

22

31

30

21

20

Durham

Falls Lake

24

Chapel Hill

19

28

WILLIAM B. UMSTEAD STATE PARK

Jordan Lake

Cary

Raleigh

Haw River

27

26

Garner

Pittsboro

25

Holly Springs

Shearon Harris Reservoir

Cape Fear River

Angier

N

| 0 | 2 | 4 | 6 miles |

| 0 | 2 | 4 | 6 kilometers |

RAVEN ROCK STATE PARK

Durham

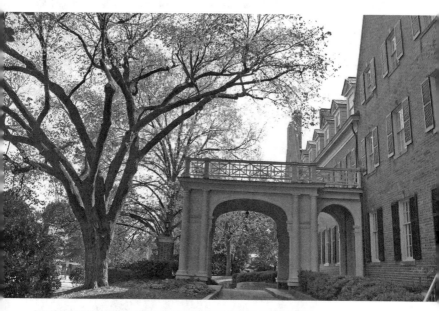

AN OAK TREE TOWERS ABOVE THE CAROLINA INN IN CHAPEL HILL.

19 Chapel Hill Franklin Street and Campus Walk

SCENERY: ★ ★ ★ ★ ★
TRAIL CONDITION: ★ ★ ★ ★ ★
CHILDREN: ★ ★ ★
DIFFICULTY: ★ ★ ★
SOLITUDE: ★

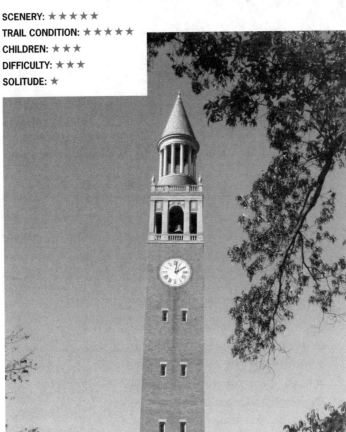

THE 14 BELLS IN THE MOREHEAD-PATTERSON BELL TOWER CHIME EACH HOUR.

GPS TRAILHEAD COORDINATES: N35° 54.614' W79° 03.797'

DISTANCE & CONFIGURATION: 2.9-mile loop

HIKING TIME: 2 hours

HIGHLIGHTS: The University of North Carolina at Chapel Hill campus, Franklin Street, bell tower, Polk Place, Kenan Memorial Stadium, and Carolina Inn

ELEVATION: 471' at trailhead to 520' at peak and 428' at lowest point

ACCESS: 24/7; free. Chapel Hill/Orange County Visitors Center (501 W. Franklin St.): Monday–Friday, 8:30 a.m.–5 p.m.; Saturday, 10 a.m.–2 p.m.

MAPS: Online at www.ci.chapel-hill.nc.us and visitchapelhill.org and at the Chapel Hill/Orange County Visitors Center, 501 W. Franklin St.

FACILITIES: None—all restrooms are connected to private businesses.

WHEELCHAIR ACCESS: Yes

COMMENTS: During school hours the campus can be extremely busy. Weekends, especially Saturdays, are an excellent time to explore this route. This is when most businesses will be open, and the campus will be less crowded.

CONTACTS: 888-968-2060; 919-968-2060; visitchapelhill.org

Overview

Chapel Hill is nicknamed the Southern Part of Heaven, and after taking a short stroll through the charming streets and brick-paved paths of the university campus, you'll find it easy to understand why. This route explores the leafy streets winding through downtown along the Franklin Street business district. Along the way you will pass historic wooded homesites, weathered stone walls, and the small shops that surround the University of North Carolina at Chapel Hill. The route follows South Columbia Street, passes the charming Carolina Inn, and turns east on Manning Drive, entering the university campus. The route through campus takes you past the main stadium and to the picturesque Morehead-Patterson Bell Tower, constructed of red brick. From here you pass the campus and walk through the main green of the campus, Polk Place, to the town's old well along East Cameron Avenue, before returning to Franklin Street and back to the visitor center.

Route Details

One of the most stunning and spectacular features of Chapel Hill is the way in which the university and the surrounding town have been masterfully integrated into the steep wooded slopes, small streams, and tree-covered vistas of the surrounding natural landscape. This artful integration has allowed the town to grow into an effective

Chapel Hill Franklin Street and Campus Walk

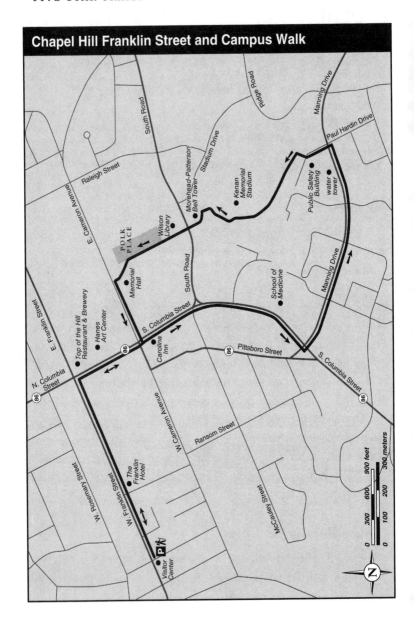

urban center while still retaining the charm and idyllic atmosphere of a small Southern town.

Chapel Hill is named after the New Hope Chapel, which stood on a hill at the crossing of East Cameron Avenue and South Columbia Street, where the Carolina Inn currently stands. The town was established in conjunction with the planning of the state's first university, and today's population of almost 49,000 consists mostly of university faculty and students. The original map of the town, drawn in 1798, shows large 2- and 4-acre lots wrapping around the northern, western, and eastern fringes of the campus that were sold at public auction to the highest bidder. The plan even proposed a 290-foot-wide "Grand Avenue" to run out of the campus through what is now Henderson Street and the Cobb Terrace area. What a sight that would be today.

Start at the Chapel Hill/Orange County Visitors Center at 501 W. Franklin St., where you can grab a map of the area. After walking out of the visitor center, turn right (northeast) and follow Franklin Street, arriving at the Franklin Hotel on your right. The Franklin opened in 2007 and helped revive the west end of Franklin Street. Selected by Fodor's as one of its top choices for hotels in the

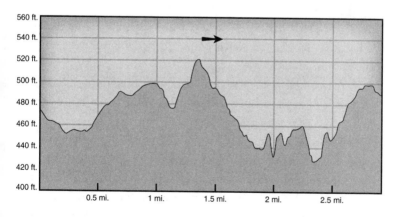

region, the Franklin lies in the heart of the college scene. Continue east on Franklin for 0.3 mile until you reach the junction with South Columbia Street. Turn right (southeast) onto Columbia Street and walk along the brick-paved path. On the left you pass a cluster of art-focused facilities, including the Ackland Art Museum and the Hanes Art Center. On the right you pass one of the many fraternity houses that are located in the downtown area.

After walking one block and crossing East Cameron Street, you arrive at the Carolina Inn. The Carolina Inn sits atop the hill where the New Hope Chapel, Chapel Hill's namesake, once stood. The elegant two-story hotel is the most famous and most popular accommodation in the Chapel Hill area. It is definitely worth going inside the hotel and exploring its lobby, a beautiful and fine example of Southern charm at its best.

After taking a brief tour of the hotel, continue along South Columbia for 0.5 mile, until you reach Manning Drive. Turn left (southeast) onto Manning and walk 0.5 mile, passing by the medical center of the university and the water tower on the left, until you reach the intersection with Paul Hardin Drive. Turn left (north) and ascend the hill, following Paul Hardin Drive for 300 feet and passing the Public Safety building on the left side, until you reach the crosswalk. Cross Paul Hardin Drive via the crosswalk and follow the redbrick path toward the Kenan Memorial Stadium, at the center of the campus.

After 200 feet you reach a split in the path. To the right a brick path leads to the north side of the stadium. Stay to the left (northwest) and continue toward the south side of the stadium through a forested section of the campus. When you reach the four-way intersection at the end of the forested section of the path, stay straight (north). Here you reach the entrance to the stadium at gate six, as well as a will-call station. Pass the entrance gate, then veer right at the stone wall and pass the south-side gates of the stadium. Oftentimes the gates to the stadium are open when there isn't an event going on, and you can walk inside and take a look around at the impressive field and stands.

Once you reach what is reportedly the world's largest ram statue, the paved brick path ends. From here, follow the paved road up the gentle hill to the north of the statue for 100 feet until you reach the stone staircase that leads to the bell tower. Follow the steps up to the circular brick path at the base of the bell tower. Turn left (west) on the circular path and follow the path around the bell tower to South Road.

Stay straight and cross South Road to continue on the brick path that leads through the campus. The path leads through Polk Place, the main green on the campus, a perfect spot for a picnic or to rest on the benches under the shade of the trees that line the green. Continue for 0.1 mile until you reach the intersection with East Cameron Avenue. Turn left (southwest) onto East Cameron and follow it for 0.1 mile until you reach the junction with South Columbia Street, where you will once again see the Carolina Inn. Turn right (northwest) onto South Columbia Street. You pass the Top of the Hill restaurant on the right, a great place to stop in for a drink or a bite to eat, and continue until you reach Franklin Street again. Turn left (southwest) and follow Franklin Street back to the visitor center, where you started.

Nearby Attractions

Restaurants, cafés, and shopping opportunities abound in the downtown Chapel Hill area. If you're going to be staying in the downtown Chapel Hill area overnight, the Carolina Inn, at 211 Pittman St., is a charming and highly recommended accommodation (800-962-8519; **carolinainn.com**). It is listed on the National Register of Historic Places and is a member of the National Trust's Historic Hotels of America.

The North Carolina Botanical Garden (see page 186) is 2.5 miles southeast of the Chapel Hill/Orange County Visitors Center. Here, you can explore more than 700 acres via paths that wind through the gardens surrounding the educational center, and you can hike the more than 2 miles of trails that meander through the nearby Piedmont forest.

Fifteen miles to the south is Jordan Lake State Park, with more than 22 miles of hiking trails spread around Jordan Lake at the Ebenezer Church Recreation Area (see page 175), New Hope Overlook (see page 169), Vista Point, Seaforth (see page 180), Parker's Creek, Crosswinds Campground, and Poplar Point Campground.

Eighteen miles east of the Chapel Hill/Orange County Visitors Center, you can visit William B. Umstead State Park (see pages 117 and 123). This 5,579-acre park offers more than 20 miles of hiking trails, as well as opportunities for paddling and boating on Big Lake, and biking and horseback riding on the bridle and biking trails. Umstead also has tent and trailer camping for $20 per day. Showers, water, and restrooms are located in the campgrounds.

Directions

From Raleigh, follow I-40 West for 15.9 miles. Merge onto NC 54 West via Exit 273A toward Chapel Hill and follow it 3.1 miles. Stay straight to go onto Raleigh Road and follow it 0.8 mile. Raleigh Road becomes South Road; follow it 0.6 mile. Turn right onto South Columbia and follow it 0.3 mile. Turn left onto West Franklin Street and follow it 0.2 mile until you reach the visitor center, on the right. If you reach Mallette Street, you've gone too far.

From Durham, take Durham Chapel Hill Boulevard and follow it 5.2 miles. After Durham Chapel Hill Boulevard becomes US 15 South, follow it 1 mile. Stay straight on East Franklin Street and follow it 3.1 miles until you reach the visitor center, on the right. If you reach Mallette Street, you've gone too far.

Downtown Durham Walk

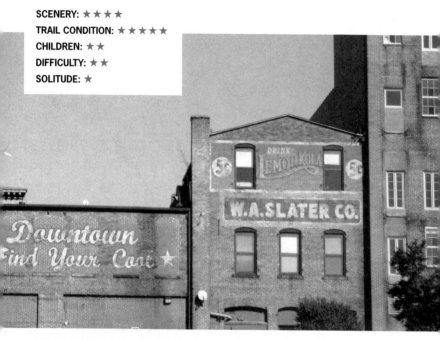

SCENERY: ★ ★ ★ ★
TRAIL CONDITION: ★ ★ ★ ★ ★
CHILDREN: ★ ★
DIFFICULTY: ★ ★
SOLITUDE: ★

THE WAREHOUSE DISTRICT OF DOWNTOWN DURHAM HAS A RUSTIC CHARM.

GPS TRAILHEAD COORDINATES: N35° 59.839' W78° 53.889'

DISTANCE & CONFIGURATION: 2.2-mile balloon

HIKING TIME: 2 hours

HIGHLIGHTS: Durham Bulls Athletic Park, Parrish Street financial district, American Tobacco District, and Warehouse District

ELEVATION: 394' at trailhead to 410' at peak and 355' at lowest point

ACCESS: 24/7; free. Durham Visitor Info Center (101 E. Morgan St.): Monday–Friday, 8:30 a.m.–5 p.m.; Saturday, 10 a.m.–2 p.m.

MAPS: Online at durham-nc.com

FACILITIES: None; all restrooms are located in private businesses.

WHEELCHAIR ACCESS: Yes

COMMENTS: Weekday mornings are excellent times to explore this route. This is when most businesses will be open and the downtown area will be less crowded.

CONTACTS: 919-687-0288; durham-nc.com

Downtown Durham Walk

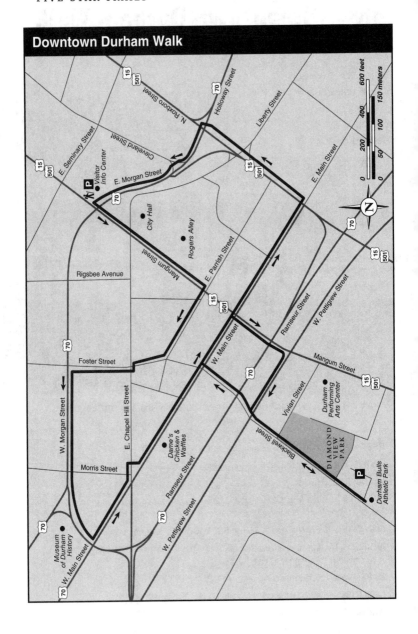

Overview

Downtown Durham is divided into several districts. This route starts at the Durham Visitor Info Center, at 101 E. Morgan St., and ventures through downtown and the main business district of the city. You pass through what is known as Black Wall Street, where African Americans established their own financial hub. From here the trail explores the Central Park District, Warehouse District, and American Tobacco District, where tobacco warehouses once occupied the majority of businesses in this area. Follow the route past the Durham Performing Arts Center to the famous Durham Bulls Athletic Park. The path returns on a mostly different route to explore more of the shopping and restaurant districts downtown before returning to the Durham Visitor Info Center.

Route Details

Park at the visitor center and get a map of the downtown area. The route starts in front of the visitor center. Walk southwest on North Mangum Street, crossing East Morgan and passing a circular fountain at the Rotary Memorial Park that is bordered with a stone wall to your left. Continue for 0.2 mile, passing the Durham City Hall and Rogers Alley on the left, until you reach West Parrish Street.

Rogers Alley is a collection of historic buildings, including the original Durham firehouse, that have been converted into shops and restaurants. Turn right (northwest) on Parrish Street. Continue for 450 feet until you reach Corcoran Street. This area of Durham is known as Black Wall Street. Six sculptures along Parrish Street mark the significance of the area and tell the story of how Durham became an African American financial center.

At the intersection of Corcoran Street, turn right (north) onto Corcoran, passing the Durham Civic Center Plaza, an outdoor park with fountains and benches, on the left. Continue for 0.2 mile until you reach the intersection with West Morgan Street. Turn left (west) onto West Morgan Street and follow it for 0.2 mile until you reach the intersection with West Main Street. Turn left (southeast) onto West Main Street, passing Dame's Chicken & Waffles on the right. Continue for 0.3 mile, passing the oldest building remaining in the downtown loop, the Queen Anne–style building at 111 W. Main St. Continue until you reach North Mangum Street. Turn right (southwest) onto North Mangum and walk 450 feet, and then turn right (northwest) onto West Pettigrew Street. Walk one block and then turn left (southwest) onto Blackwell Street, passing on your right the Old Bull Building, one of the nation's oldest tobacco warehouses, which has been restored and turned into apartments.

Continue for 0.2 mile, passing on the left the impressive Durham Performing Arts Center and the expansive green in front of the interesting building. The arts center holds 2,800 people, making it the largest in the Carolinas, and it has the largest stage between Atlanta and Washington, D.C. After passing the arts center you reach the famous Durham Bulls Athletic Park, the 10,000-seat stadium for the 2009 AAA Baseball National Champions, the Durham Bulls.

From here turn around and backtrack to the intersection of West Main Street, 0.2 mile away. Turn right (southeast) and continue on West Main Street for 0.2 mile until you reach North Roxboro Street. Turn left (northeast) onto North Roxboro Street and follow it for 0.2 mile until you reach East Morgan Street. Turn left (northwest), following East Morgan for 0.2 mile until you return to the visitor center.

Nearby Attractions

The Al Buehler Cross Country Trail at Duke University (see page 144) is 4 miles to the northwest. The 4-mile walking and running trail is a great way to explore the Duke University campus and the surrounding forested areas. Also in the same area near the campus, only 3 miles to the northwest of downtown Durham, are the Sarah P. Duke Gardens (see page 198). The 55-acre gardens, in the West Campus adjacent to Duke University Medical Center, can be explored free of charge.

Considered one of the premier gardens in the United States, it hosts more than 300,000 visitors a year. If you are staying in the Durham area, the Washington Duke Inn is on the Duke University campus and is highly recommended. Built in the style of an English country inn, the hotel is home to the Duke University Golf Course.

Directions

From Raleigh, take I-40 West and follow it for 9 miles. Merge onto NC 147 North via Exit 279B toward Durham/Downtown and follow it 7.4 miles. Take Exit 12B toward US 15-BR/Downtown. Stay straight to go onto Jackie Robinson Drive and follow it 0.1 mile. Turn right onto South Roxboro Street and follow it 0.5 mile. Turn left onto Holloway Street and follow it 0.2 mile until you reach the Durham Visitor Info Center, on the right at 101 E. Morgan St.

In Durham, the visitor center is at the intersection of West Morgan and North Mangum Streets.

21

Duke University:
Al Buehler Cross Country Trail

SCENERY: ★ ★ ★ ★
TRAIL CONDITION: ★ ★ ★ ★ ★
CHILDREN: ★ ★ ★ ★ ★
DIFFICULTY: ★ ★ ★
SOLITUDE: ★

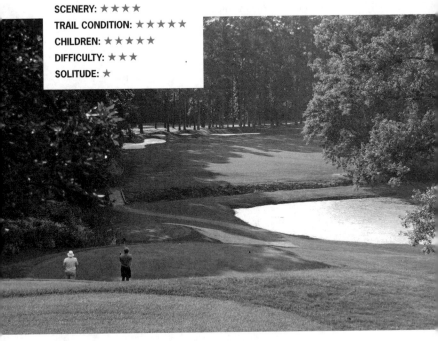

THE CROSS-COUNTRY TRAIL CIRCLES THE DUKE UNIVERSITY GOLF COURSE.

GPS TRAILHEAD COORDINATES: N35° 59.523' W78° 56.810'

DISTANCE & CONFIGURATION: 2.8-mile loop

HIKING TIME: 1.5 hours

HIGHLIGHTS: Washington Duke Inn and Duke Golf Course

ELEVATION: 353' at trailhead to 400' at peak and 274' at lowest point

ACCESS: 24/7; free

MAPS: Online at www.dukeforest.duke.edu and at the Cross Country Trailhead. Detailed maps of the entire Duke Forest can be purchased at the Office of the Duke Forest.

FACILITIES: Restrooms, water fountains, and emergency phones

WHEELCHAIR ACCESS: None

COMMENTS: This is a popular trail with cross-country runners—be alert and give them the right-of-way. To avoid crowds, visit late mornings during the week.

CONTACTS: 919-613-8013; www.dukeforest.duke.edu

Overview

Explore the grounds of the Duke University campus on this mostly gravel cross-country trail that winds through the forest surrounding the Washington Duke Inn and golf course. Adjacent to the Duke Forest, this cross-country trail is a perfect choice for runners and walkers. The route follows the Al Buehler Cross Country Trail main loop and starts from the main parking lot, just off Cameron Boulevard near the junction with University Boulevard. The trail is extremely popular, and the parking lot fills easily. Another lot is farther down Cameron Boulevard to the west, just past the business school. Venture through the forest and across winding streams before heading south as the path follows alongside the US 15-501 Bypass. Throughout the trail you will get glimpses of long expanses of the golf course; you may even have the opportunity to judge golfers' swings as you walk along the trail circling the impressive course.

Route Details

Start your hike from the main parking lot along Cameron Boulevard. From the south side of the parking lot, follow the thin gravel path to the larger, main gravel trail—the Al Buehler Cross Country Trail. The path is very well maintained and easy to follow; however, many of the junctions are poorly marked or not marked at all. If you do get turned around while you are on the trail, you will most likely be able to ask someone who is walking the trail which way to go. This is an extremely popular trail with students and area residents. You are likely to see teams of runners and individuals training. Please be courteous and give these athletes the right-of-way. This is a campus facility, and therefore the main focus of the trail is to provide university athletes with a training ground.

The cross-country trail on which you are walking is named after Al Buehler, who coached 10 All-Americans, seven Penn Relay champions, six Atlantic Coast Conference championship cross-country teams, and five Olympians. Two of these Olympians went on to win

Duke University: Al Buehler Cross Country Trail

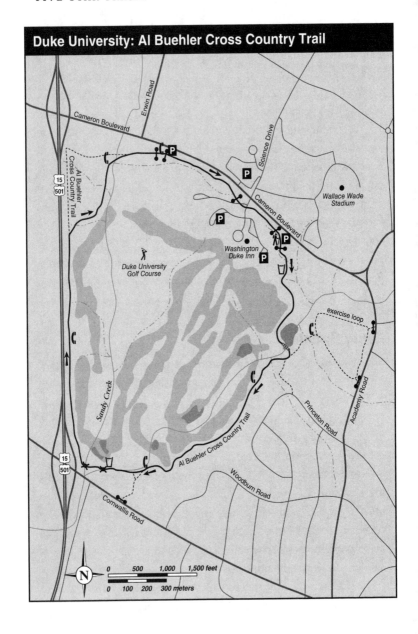

medals. In 1972, 1984, and 1988 Buehler served as team manager for the US Olympic track and field teams in Los Angeles; Munich, Germany; and Seoul, South Korea, respectively.

Once you reach the main trail, turn left (south) onto the shaded gravel path that leads into the forest. Mile markers are posted along the way to measure your progress as you walk. After 0.1 mile you come to a boardwalk that crosses several streams and a surrounding wetland area. Continue on the main trail for 0.2 mile until you reach a wetland retention pond on your left. About 150 feet from the retention pond, you will reach an unmarked junction in the trail. To the left, a spur trail leads to the exercise loop. If you want to extend the length of your walk, take the spur trail to the exercise loop, where you will find sit-up benches, chin-up bars, and stretching centers. To stay on the main trail, turn right (southwest).

From here the trail is very easy to follow. The trail goes over small hills that add a bit of challenge to your walk. Here and there the trail comes right up to the golf course that the trail circles. After 0.7 mile you reach two spur trails to your left (south) that are very close to one another, and both lead to Cornwallis Road. Stay

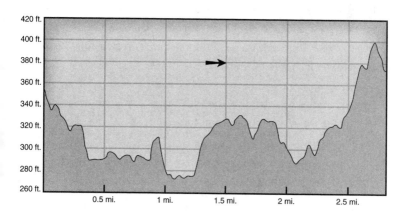

straight (west) on the main path. After an additional 0.2 mile, the trail turns to the right as you start to circle around and head toward the north. You cross several streams as the trail follows alongside the US 15-501 Bypass, but the trail is far enough away from the road that you hardly ever hear road noise. After 0.6 mile walking in this northerly direction, the trail curves to the right and begins heading toward the east. After walking 0.4 mile you reach a parking lot to your left. The trail skirts the edge of the parking lot and continues to follow alongside Cameron Boulevard. Continue for 0.3 mile until you reach Faculty Club Drive. The trail continues straight ahead (east). To the right (south), Faculty Club Drive leads to the Washington Duke Inn.

If you want to make a night of your trip to the Duke campus, there is no better place to stay than the Washington Duke Inn (3001 Cameron Blvd.; 800-443-3853; **washingtondukeinn.com**). Built in the style of an English country manor, the inn is nestled into 300 acres of forest and golf course. Inside, elegant furnishings and spacious guestrooms match the impressive exterior. Named after an American tobacco industrialist and the owner of W. Duke Sons Tobacco Company, the inn is an institution on campus that commemorates the university's largest sole benefactor. George Washington Duke was responsible for moving Duke University, then known as Trinity College, to Durham. He was also responsible for convincing the college to open its doors to women.

Stay straight (southeast) and cross Faculty Club Drive, continuing on the main trail. After walking 0.1 mile you reach the parking lot where you started and the end of the Al Buehler Cross Country Trail.

Nearby Attractions

Spread out around the Duke University campus is Duke Forest, 7,020 acres of land in Alamance, Durham, and Orange Counties that is broken up into six separate forest areas. There are more than 5 miles of hiking trails to explore in the Duke Forest, including the popular 0.8-mile Shepherd Nature Trail off of NC 751 at Gate C.

Just 4 miles to the east of the Al Buehler Cross Country Trail is downtown Durham (see page 139). You can explore many of the highlights in the downtown district, including the Durham Bulls Athletic Park, the Parrish Street financial district, and the American Tobacco and Warehouse Districts. Distinguished as one of the major hubs of tobacco distribution in the 1900s, as well as a financial capital for African Americans, downtown Durham today is experiencing a renaissance, with many of the spacious tobacco warehouses being transformed into lofty apartment buildings, restaurants, and shopping plazas. Experience the local flavor at Dame's Chicken and Waffles, or grab a hot dog and a box of Cracker Jacks and dig into a taste of Americana tradition with the Durham Bulls, America's most famous AAA baseball team.

Stop by the Sarah P. Duke Gardens (see page 198), just 1 mile east of the Al Buehler Cross Country Trail. The 55-acre garden is in the west campus, adjacent to Duke University Medical Center. There is no charge to enjoy the colorful and lush landscape, considered one of the premier gardens in the United States; it hosts more than 300,000 visitors a year.

Directions

From Raleigh, the Al Buehler Cross Country Trail is 25 miles to the northwest. Take Wade Avenue to I-40 West and follow I-40 for 9 miles. Merge onto NC 147 North via Exit 279B toward Durham/Downtown and follow it 9.7 miles. Take the Elba Street/Trent Drive exit, Exit 15A, and keep left to take the Trent Drive ramp. Turn left onto Trent Drive and follow it 0.1 mile. Turn right onto Erwin Road and follow it 0.4 mile. Turn left onto Research Drive, pass through one roundabout, and follow the road 0.3 mile. You will reach the parking lot to the Al Buehler Cross Country Trail straight ahead. If you reach Coal Pile Drive, you've gone too far.

From Durham, take NC 147 North to the Elba Street/Trent Drive exit, Exit 15A, and follow it 0.3 mile. Keep left to take the Trent Drive ramp. Turn left onto Trent Drive and follow it 0.1 mile. Turn right onto Erwin Road and follow it 0.4 mile. Turn left onto Research Drive, pass through one roundabout, and follow the road 0.3 mile. You will reach the parking lot to the Al Buehler Cross Country Trail straight ahead. If you reach Coal Pile Drive, you've gone too far.

Eno River State Park:
Bobbitt Hole Trail

SCENERY: ★ ★ ★ ★ ★
TRAIL CONDITION: ★ ★ ★ ★ ★
CHILDREN: ★ ★ ★ ★
DIFFICULTY: ★ ★ ★
SOLITUDE: ★ ★

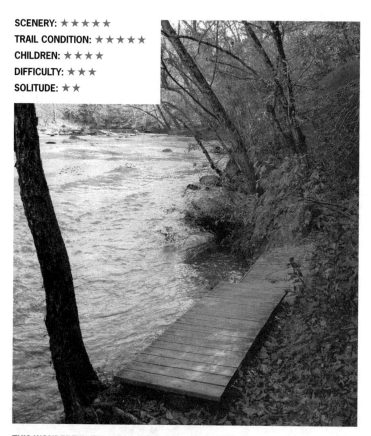

THIS WONDERFUL TRAIL FOLLOWS ALONG THE ENO RIVER.

GPS TRAILHEAD COORDINATES: N36° 03.463' W78° 58.817'

DISTANCE & CONFIGURATION: 2.4-mile loop

HIKING TIME: 2 hours

HIGHLIGHTS: Bobbitt Hole, Eno River, rock formations, and bluffs

ELEVATION: 400' at trailhead to 478' at peak and 346' at lowest point

ACCESS: November–February: Daily, 9 a.m.–5:30 p.m. March–April and September–October: Daily, 9 a.m.–7:30 p.m. May–August: Daily, 9 a.m.–8:30 p.m. Free; campsites $13/day.

Eno River State Park: Bobbitt Hole Trail

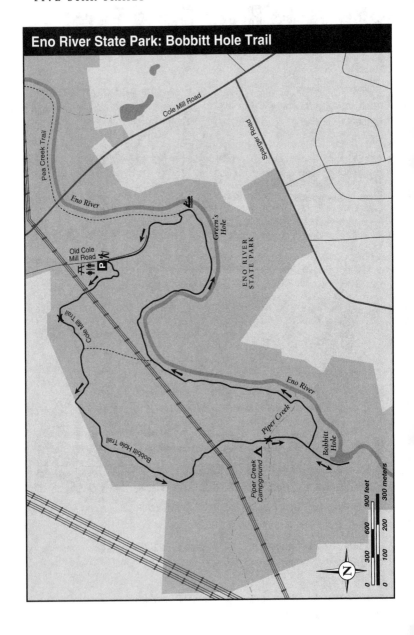

MAPS: Online at ncparks.gov, at the park office, and at the trailhead kiosk

FACILITIES: Restrooms, picnic tables, water fountain, canoe and kayak launch, and backcountry campsites

WHEELCHAIR ACCESS: None, but a short paved trail that leads from the trailhead to the picnic area is wheelchair-accessible.

COMMENTS: Eno River State Park has several recreation areas, and they all have different operating hours. If you would like to visit several areas of the state park in one trip, check the operating hours ahead of time. Pets are allowed on the trail as long as they are on leashes no longer than 6 feet.

CONTACTS: 919-383-1686; ncparks.gov

Overview

This trail leads to the Bobbitt Hole, one of the most scenic areas along the Eno River. At Bobbitt Hole a rock outcrop towers over the river on the south bank, where a small cascade drops into an 18-feet-deep hole before the river turns sharply to the east. The Bobbitt Hole Trail starts in the parking lot of the Cole Mill area in the eastern side of the park. From here the trail leads to the Bobbitt Hole and the Eno River, traversing through the forest and over several hills and drainages. The trail turns sharply to the east and follows along the bank of the

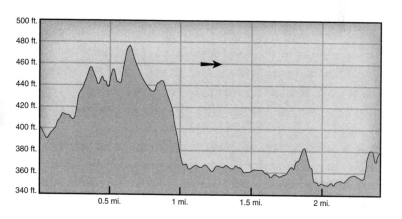

Eno River, shaded with trees along the route, before heading uphill and returning to the parking lot at the end of the loop.

Route Details

Follow Old Cole Mill Road to the eastern entrance of the park, and leave your vehicle at the first lot on the right side. The trailhead is directly in front of the parking lot. The beginning of the trail is rather confusing, and the maps you get from the park visitor center do not help clarify what way you should go to get to the Bobbitt Hole Trail. The signs or blazes during the beginning section of the trail don't help much either. This beginning section is like a maze of spur trails, and the easiest way to get to the Bobbitt Hole Trail is to turn left at the first split in the trail, follow it for 60 feet, and then turn right onto the Brown Trail, which leads toward the Bobbitt Hole Trail. Continue for 50 feet until you reach an intersection in the trail, and turn right (northwest) toward the Bobbitt Hole Trail.

Continue on the spur trail for 0.2 mile until the trail crosses a creek via a small wooden footbridge. From here the trail ascends for 400 feet to a split in the trail. Turn right (west) onto the Bobbitt Hole Trail, which is blazed with red dots, and continue for 0.6 mile, passing through a clearing made for power lines and reaching the Piper Creek Campground. Restrooms are available at Piper Creek Campground; at the park office, you can reserve a spot to camp.

The trail descends for 0.3 mile, crossing over Piper Creek on a short wooden bridge and heading toward the impressive Bobbitt Hole. During the weekends and holidays, when the trails are busy, a small group of people will usually be admiring the scenic view from the clearing along the riverbank and relaxing on the benches that line Bobbitt Hole. Beavers, some of the most curious and interesting creatures to inhabit the river, can often be seen along the next stretch of trail, which leads from the Bobbitt Hole and follows along the Eno River. These resilient animals were almost killed off in North Carolina due to excessive trapping but have now returned to many parts of the state.

They are most active at night and are seldom seen during the day. The best times to see beavers along the Bobbitt Hole Trail are during the early morning and at dusk. Gnawed-off stumps and tree trunks are telltale signs that a beaver has been searching for food in the area.

More than 100 kinds of songbirds are found on the Eno River. The calls of the red-tailed hawk, barred owl, and crows can also be heard in the park. Around the river, look for wood ducks, great blue herons, and belted kingfishers. In the forest, wild turkeys, white-tailed deer, raccoons, squirrels, chipmunks, and opossums feed on the fruits and seeds of the hardwood forest. More elusive are the otters and bobcats that inhabit the park.

Spend some time exploring Bobbitt Hole and enjoying the view of the river, with the towering rock formations on the south bank. Then turn around and follow the spur trail back to the Bobbitt Hole Trail; turn right (east) and continue on the Bobbitt Hole Trail, which follows alongside the Eno River. After following the river for 0.5 mile, you reach a split in the trail. To the left, an unmarked trail leads uphill and reconnects with the northern side of the Cole Mill Trail. However, stay straight (east) on the Bobbitt Hole Trail and continue along the river. After 0.1 mile the trail curves around to the right (south), follows the riverbank for 0.2 mile, and then turns sharply to the left (north) and leaves the river behind.

Continue uphill for 400 feet, walking away from the river, until you come to a staircase leading to a picnic area. Stay straight (north) and continue on the Bobbitt Hole Trail for 500 feet, where you pass the canoe and kayak launch on the riverbank to your right, and climb uphill to reach the parking lot and trailhead. From here you just have to follow the road through the parking lot to return to your vehicle, which is parked in the first lot 90 feet away.

Nearby Attractions

Eno River State Park (also see page 157) has more than 24 miles of hiking trails to explore. The 190-acre Occoneechee Mountain State

Natural Area (see page 192), 10 miles southwest of Eno River State Park, offers more than 4 miles of hiking trails.

Eight miles east of Eno River is West Point on the Eno (see page 204), a 388-acre Durham city park with more than 3 miles of hiking trails that further explore the Eno River and the surrounding forest. Within the park, take a tour of a replica of the original West Point Mill and buy some fresh stone-ground flour and cornmeal, which are made on-site. Swimming and fishing are very popular in the park as well.

Directions

Eno River State Park is 12 miles northwest of Durham, and the drive usually takes about 20 minutes. From Durham, take I-85 South and merge onto US 70 West at Exit 170; follow US 70 for 0.5 mile. Take the first right onto Pleasant Green Road and follow it 2.2 miles. Turn right onto Cole Mill Road and follow it 1.2 miles. Turn right onto Old Cole Mill Road and follow it until you reach the Cole Mill parking lot and the Bobbitt Hole Trailhead, on the right.

23

Eno River State Park:
Cox Mountain Trail

SCENERY: ★ ★ ★ ★ ★
TRAIL CONDITION: ★ ★ ★ ★ ★
CHILDREN: ★ ★
DIFFICULTY: ★ ★ ★ ★ ★
SOLITUDE: ★ ★

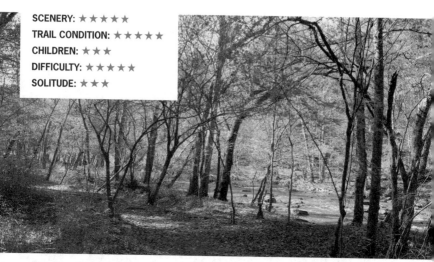

IF YOU'RE LOOKING FOR A CHALLENGE, THEN HIKE THE COX MOUNTAIN TRAIL.

GPS TRAILHEAD COORDINATES: N36° 04.430' W79° 00.380'

DISTANCE & CONFIGURATION: 4.2-mile balloon

HIKING TIME: 3 hours

HIGHLIGHTS: Cox Mountain, Eno River, and suspension bridge

ELEVATION: 459' at trailhead to 668' at peak and 400' at lowest point

ACCESS: November–February: Daily, 8 a.m.–6 p.m. March–April and September–October: Daily, 8 a.m.–8 p.m. May–August: Daily, 8 a.m.–9 p.m. Free.

MAPS: Online at ncparks.gov, at the park office, and at the trailhead kiosk

FACILITIES: Restrooms, picnic tables, water fountain, canoe and kayak launch, and backcountry campsites

WHEELCHAIR ACCESS: None on this trail, but a short paved trail leading from the trailhead to the picnic area is wheelchair-accessible.

COMMENTS: Eno River State Park has several recreation areas, and they all have different operating hours. If you would like to visit several areas of the state park in one trip, check the operating hours ahead of time. This hike is fairly challenging for the area, so be prepared for a challenging climb. Pets are allowed on the trail as long as they are on leashes no longer than 6 feet.

CONTACTS: 919-383-1686; ncparks.gov

Eno River State Park: Cox Mountain Trail

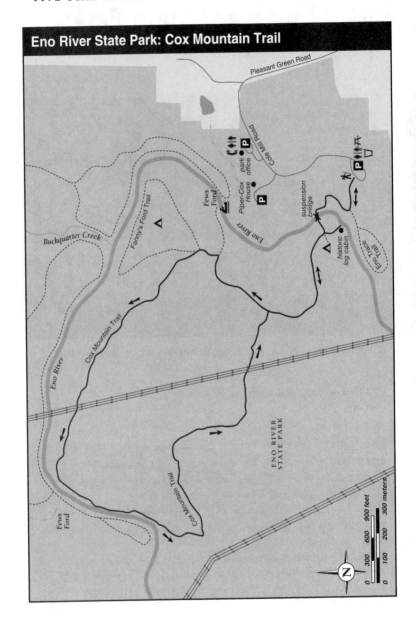

Overview

Eno River State Park creates a 3,900-acre protective forest corridor that surrounds the winding banks of the Eno River. The Eno flows from northwest Orange County into Durham County for 33 miles, where it joins the Flat River to become the Neuse and flows into Falls Lake. The state park is 12 miles northwest of the city of Durham and just minutes from Chapel Hill and Hillsborough, making it an exceptionally popular destination for outdoor recreation in the warmer months of spring, summer, and fall.

The Cox Mountain Trail is exceptionally challenging for this area, where most of the trails are mostly moderate to easy, yet the trail is definitely worth the workout. Starting from the Fews Ford Picnic Area, the trail descends to the Eno River and crosses the river on a suspension bridge. The trail follows the old Hillsborough Coach Road before going over the top of Cox Mountain and then gradually descending to the riverbank. You cross the suspension bridge again, which offers excellent views of the river, and return to the parking lot at Fews Ford where you began.

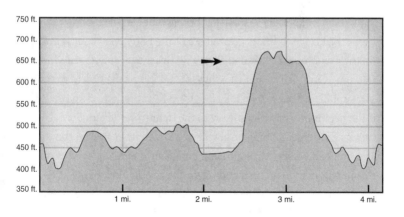

Route Details

Cox Mountain Trail starts from the western side of the parking lot. The trail is clearly marked with a brown sign, and a paved path leads past a kiosk where you can also find maps of this particular section of the park. To the right are water fountains and a spur trail that leads to a picnic area. Continue past the spur trail. The paved trail ends and a 3-foot-wide unpaved trail, blazed with blue dots, enters into the forest.

In the forest surrounding the Eno River, what farming and the timber industry once took away has been given the opportunity to grow through the preservation action of the state park, and the ridges, slopes, and floodplains are once again thick with vegetation. In the upland forests, oak, beech, poplar, maple, dogwood, pine, and hickory trees dominate. Along the riverbanks you find sycamore, birch, and hornbeam trees. On the slopes of the steep bluffs you will see the hardy mountain laurels, Catawba rhododendrons, and ferns growing. If you want to catch wildflowers blooming in the fields and forest, visit the area February–November.

After 500 feet you reach the junction with the Eno Trace Trail. Stay straight (northeast) and continue on the Cox Mountain Trail, which leads down a series of small steps and follows along the riverbank to an impressive suspension bridge that crosses the Eno River. Cross the bridge (it offers great views of the Eno River) and continue on the Cox Mountain Trail until you reach a junction with the Group Camping Trail. Turn right (northwest) and follow the Cox Mountain Trail uphill and over small hills for 0.4 mile until the trail splits. This is the beginning of the loop. Stay to the right toward Fews Ford. Hike for an additional 0.2 mile until you come to another split in the trail. The trail can be slightly confusing here, and it is really easy to miss this junction and end up standing on the riverbank, looking at Fews Ford and wondering where you are. If you make it to Fews Ford, you've gone too far and need to turn around.

At the split in the trail, turn left (north) toward the Fanny's Ford Trail and continue uphill for 230 feet until you reach a three-way split in the trail. To the right (northeast), Fanny's Ford Trail leads toward the riverbank to a backcountry campsite that is marked on the park map. If you stay straight (north), you take the other side of the Fanny's Ford Trail that leads to the same place. However, stay all the way to the left (northwest) and continue on the blue-dot-blazed Cox Mountain Trail, which begins the gradual ascent to the top of Cox Mountain.

The next 0.6 mile begins the challenging section of this trail. From here you climb up to a clearing that runs beneath power lines close to the top of Cox Mountain. You don't actually reach the top of Cox Mountain until you circle back around on the loop trail and climb the mountain again, but over this 0.6 mile you climb more than 400 feet in elevation. It's a gradual climb but challenging nonetheless. From here it's a slightly steeper 0.4-mile descent of the mountain until you reach the riverbank. The riverbank along this section is exceedingly pleasant, lined with remarkably beautiful trees and dotted with large boulders.

The trail follows alongside the riverbank and turns sharply to the left (west). The path is very well marked with signs and blazes, and this sharp turn is easy to follow. The trail then begins another ascent, this one a mile long and gradual at first and then very steep at the end. During this second ascension to the top of Cox Mountain, you climb more than 500 feet and reach the highest elevation on the trail. The clearing atop Cox Mountain is accompanied by the power lines, but the area here offers great views of the surrounding rolling hills. This is a really nice spot to take a break and enjoy the vista after the long climb uphill.

Continue on the Cox Mountain Trail for 0.2 mile and begin the descent of the mountain to a junction with the Group Camping Trail. Turn right (south) and continue 20 feet to a spur trail on the right side of the trail that leads to a really interesting historical cabin on the riverbank. This is an optional side trip, but I highly recommend it. The idyllic setting of the cabin on the riverbank can make you want to stay forever. The picnic table in front of the cabin makes a great spot to stop for lunch or a snack. There's even a cell-phone audio tour for the cabin. Just dial the number on the plaque in front of the cabin, and you'll hear a prerecorded interpretive program about the site. After exploring the cabin, follow the Cox Mountain Trail for 0.3 mile back across the suspension bridge and out to the parking lot and trailhead.

Nearby Attractions

Eno River State Park has more than 24 miles of hiking trails to explore. One of the most scenic areas along the Eno River is Bobbitt Hole (see page 151), which can be reached by walking the 1.7-mile Bobbitt Hole Trail. The 190-acre Occoneechee Mountain State Natural Area (see page 192), 10 miles southwest of Eno River State Park, offers more than 4 miles of hiking trails.

Eight miles east of Eno River is West Point on the Eno (see page 204), a 388-acre Durham city park with more than 3 miles of hiking trails that further explore the Eno River and the surrounding forest. Within the park, take a tour of a replica of the original West Point Mill and buy some fresh stone-ground flour and cornmeal, which are made on-site. Swimming and fishing are very popular in the park as well.

Directions

Eno River State Park is 12 miles northwest of Durham, and the drive usually takes about 20 minutes. From Durham, take I-85 South and merge onto US 70 West at Exit 170; follow US 70 for 0.5 mile. Take the first right onto Pleasant Green Road and follow it 2.2 miles. Turn left onto Cole Mill Road and follow it 1 mile until Cole Mill Road ends at the park's Fews Ford Access, on the left.

24

Falls Lake State Recreation Area:

B. W. Wells Recreation Area

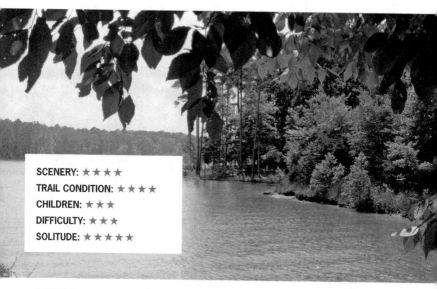

SCENERY: ★ ★ ★ ★
TRAIL CONDITION: ★ ★ ★ ★
CHILDREN: ★ ★ ★
DIFFICULTY: ★ ★ ★
SOLITUDE: ★ ★ ★ ★ ★

A VISTA OF FALLS LAKE FROM THE TRAIL

GPS TRAILHEAD COORDINATES: N35° 59.418' W78° 37.983'

DISTANCE & CONFIGURATION: 1.9-mile loop

HIKING TIME: 1 hour

HIGHLIGHTS: Falls Lake

ELEVATION: 322' at trailhead to 362' at peak and 250' at lowest point

ACCESS: November–February: Daily, 8 a.m.–6 p.m. March–April and September–October: Daily, 8 a.m.–8 p.m. May–August: Daily, 8 a.m.–9 p.m.; closed December 25. Cars, $6/day; seniors age 62 and older, $4/day; annual pass, $50.

MAPS: Online at ncparks.gov, at the park's visitor center, or at the trailhead kiosk

FACILITIES: Restrooms, picnic facilities, pavilions, boat launch, marina, and fishing pier

WHEELCHAIR ACCESS: None on this trail. However, many park activities—including the fishing piers at Beaverdam and Rollingview and picnic shelters at Beaverdam, Rolling View, and Sandling Beach—can be accessed by persons in wheelchairs. Accessible campsites are available at Holly Point, Rolling View, and Shinleaf.

CONTACTS: 919-676-1027; ncparks.gov

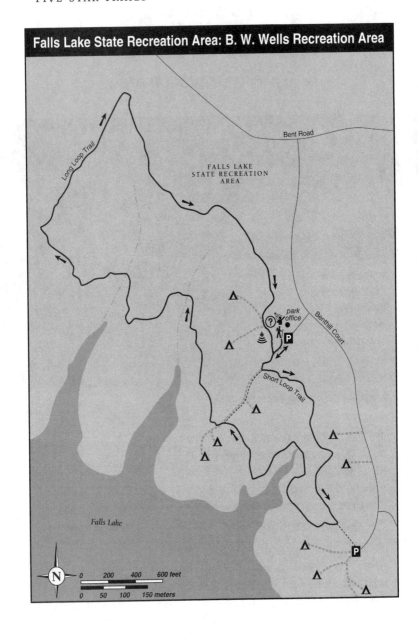

Falls Lake State Recreation Area: B. W. Wells Recreation Area

FALLS LAKE
STATE RECREATION
AREA

Bent Road

Long Loop Trail

park
office

Benthill Court

Short Loop Trail

Falls Lake

0   200   400   600 feet

0   50   100   150 meters

N

Overview

This route explores the B. W. Wells Recreation Area, combining the Long Loop Trail and the Short Loop Trail. The path begins from the trailhead in the first parking lot on the west side of Benthill Court. The trail ventures along the shore of Falls Lake, briefly offering incredible views of the lake as you walk. After leaving the lakeshore, the trail loops through the forest before returning to the trailhead. Along the route you pass several group campsites. This is a sparsely used portion of the Falls Lake Recreation Area. If you're searching for some solitude, then you've come to the right place. For this reason, the hike is one of my favorites.

Route Details

Oaks and loblolly pines dominate the forest surrounding Falls Lake. A wide variety of wildflowers, including butterfly weeds, tickseed sunflowers, and asters, can be seen blooming throughout the forests. During the day you are likely to spot white-tailed deer, rabbits, and possibly red foxes in the forest. While hiking along the lakeshore, keep an eye out for the wood ducks and mallards that inhabit

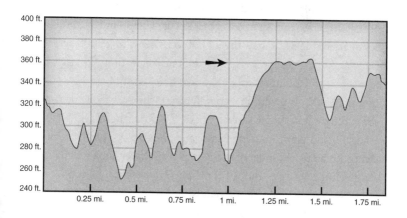

the lake. You might spot diving ospreys, bald eagles, and red-tailed hawks as they search to sink their talons into the abundant fish found in the lake's waters. More elusive are the great horned owls, barred owls, screech owls, and raccoons that are heard and seen in the forest at night.

On the west side of the parking lot you will find a small path that runs north into the forest. The only signage to guide you toward the trailhead for the Short Loop Trail is a sign for campsites 3, 4, and 5. Follow these signs and head west on a thin spur trail into the forest for 100 feet until you reach a kiosk and the official trailhead for the Short Loop Trail. At this kiosk stay straight (west) and walk another 100 feet until you reach a trail junction. Here, facing the kiosk, the Long Loop Trail is behind you to the north. Turn left (south) onto the Short Loop Trail, passing an open field on the left. Walk 0.3 mile until you reach a split in the trail. To the left a spur trail leads to a parking lot at the southern end of Benthill Court. Turn right (southwest) and continue on the Short Loop Trail toward the shore of Falls Lake. After 0.1 mile you will reach Falls Lake.

Another inventive project by the US Army Corps of Engineers, the Falls Lake Dam was constructed to prevent the all-too-common catastrophic flooding that occurred along the banks of the Neuse River. The project to construct the dam began in 1978 and was completed in 1981. Today, the 12,000-acre lake and 26,000 acres of woodlands that comprise Falls Lake State Recreation Area provide recreation and hunting opportunities, flood control, and a source of water for the surrounding communities. The park is divided into seven different sections: Beaverdam, B. W. Wells, Highway 50, Holly Point, Rolling View, Sandling Beach, and Shinleaf. The park has more than 300 campsites, most with electricity and water hookups that are suitable for both tent and RV campers. Showers and restrooms are available in each of the campgrounds.

Continue on the Short Loop Trail for 0.2 mile, zigzagging your way along the shore of the lake until you reach a gravel road. Cross the road, and on the other side you will reach a junction with the Long

Loop Trail. Stay straight and join the white-blazed Long Loop Trail. Continue along the lakeshore for 0.5 mile. The trail here turns sharply to the right (northeast). Stay on the white-blazed Long Loop Trail for 0.2 mile, walking through the forest, until you reach another sharp turn to the right (south). Stay on the Long Loop Trail for 0.4 mile more, heading south, until you reach the gravel road again. Turn left (west) on the gravel road toward the restrooms in front of you. After 75 feet you will reach the parking lot where you started the trail.

Nearby Attractions

Falls Lake State Recreation Area offers more than 20 miles of hiking trails, including a portion of the Mountains-to-Sea Trail that traverses the south shore of the lake, as well as other shorter trails at Beaver Dam, B. W. Wells, Holly Point, Rolling View, and Sandling Beach.

Blue Jay Point County Park (see page 26), a 236-acre park on the shores of Falls Lake in northern Wake County, offers more than 5 miles of trails within its boundaries, as well as open play fields, playgrounds, an environmental-education center, and an overnight lodge. The park features hiking trails that also connect with the Falls Lake State Recreation Area trails to offer longer hiking opportunities. The park is 5 miles south of Falls Lake State Recreation Area.

William B. Umstead State Park (see pages 117 and 123) is 13 miles south of Falls Lake State Recreation Area. This 5,579-acre park offers more than 20 miles of hiking trails, as well as opportunities for paddling and boating on Big Lake, and biking and horseback riding on the bridle and biking trails throughout the park. Umstead also has tent and trailer camping for $20 per day. Showers, water, and restrooms are available in the campgrounds.

Directions

From Raleigh, head northwest on Glenwood Avenue/US 70 East until you reach Creedmoor Road/NC 50 North. Turn right onto Creedmoor Road/NC 50 North and follow it 11.7 miles. The entrance to Falls Lake State Recreation Area will be on your right. If you reach Easy Horse Trail, you've gone too far.

From Durham, start out by going east on Holloway Street/US 70 and follow it for 12.3 miles until you reach Creedmoor Road/NC 50 North. Merge onto Creedmoor Road/NC 50 North and follow it 2 miles. The entrance to Falls Lake State Recreation Area will be on your right. If you reach Easy Horse Trail, you've gone too far.

25

Jordan Lake State Recreation Area: Blue Trail

SCENERY: ★ ★ ★ ★ ★
TRAIL CONDITION: ★ ★ ★ ★
CHILDREN: ★ ★ ★
DIFFICULTY: ★ ★ ★ ★
SOLITUDE: ★ ★ ★ ★

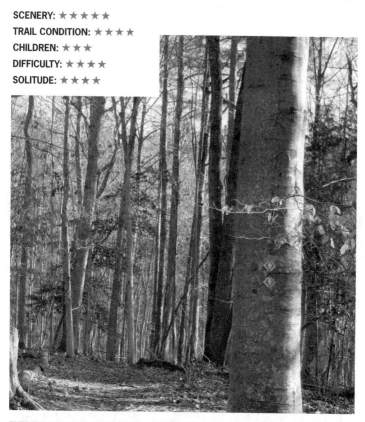

EXPLORE THE FOREST AND THE LAKE ALONG THIS HILLY TRAIL.

GPS TRAILHEAD COORDINATES: N35° 40.948' W79° 02.878'

DISTANCE & CONFIGURATION: 2.6-mile loop

HIKING TIME: 2 hours

HIGHLIGHTS: Jordan Lake, hardwood forest, and creeks

ELEVATION: 240' at trailhead to 355' at peak

ACCESS: May–August: Daily, 8 a.m.–9 p.m.; September–October and March–April: Daily, 8 a.m.–8 p.m.; November–February: Daily, 8 a.m.–6 p.m.; closed December 25. Memorial Day–Labor Day: daily, $6 admission; April–May and September on weekends and holidays: $6 admission; otherwise free.

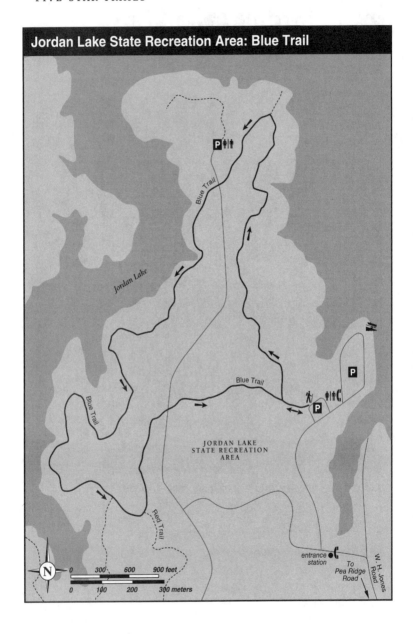

Jordan Lake State Recreation Area: Blue Trail

MAPS: Online at ncparks.gov, at the park's visitor center, and at the trailhead kiosk

FACILITIES: Boat ramp, restrooms, and water fountains

WHEELCHAIR ACCESS: No

COMMENTS: This park is very popular in the summer, when the boating crowd arrives to enjoy the 14,000 acres of water in the reservoir. The trails are heavily used on holidays and weekends, especially in the summer. The best time to enjoy the park is on weekdays during the spring and fall, which are also coincidentally the seasons in which the weather is best suited for hiking. Dogs are welcome on the trails as long as they are well behaved and kept on leashes no longer than 6 feet.

CONTACTS: 919-362-0586; ncparks.gov

Overview

The 14,000-acre park has more than 22 miles of hiking trails, and the New Hope Overlook area is on the southwest side of the park near Moncure, North Carolina. The New Hope Overlook area has two trails, the Red Trail and the Blue Trail. This hike follows the Blue Trail, which offers excellent views of Jordan Lake. The route traverses a mature hardwood forest and crosses several tributary creeks, climbing over a couple of hills in the beginning of the trail and climaxing with a challenging climb of an exceptionally steep hill at the very end of the trail.

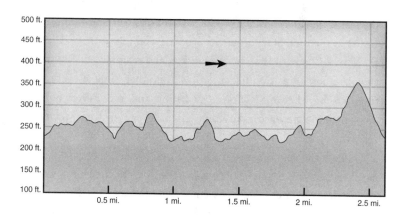

Route Details

Settled by Scottish Highlanders in the 1740s and inhabited for more than 10,000 years by American Indians, the New Hope River Valley has been utilized by a great range of cultures. Battles of the Civil and Revolutionary Wars were fought in this area, but today the landscape is much different than what the soldiers and peoples of the past would have recognized. The US Army Corps of Engineers built the dam that made it possible to flood the valley and create the 13,000-acre reservoir. Plans to build the dam were first submitted to the US House of Representatives in 1933, and nearly 50 years later in 1981 the valley was flooded and Jordan Lake was created, the name honoring B. Everett Jordan, a former senator from North Carolina. The surrounding park conserves more than 32,000 acres of the New Hope River Valley for recreation and wildlife management.

The Blue Trail starts from the New Hope Overlook parking lot. The kiosk and trailhead are in the northwest corner of the lot. Follow the 4-foot-wide unpaved path, marked with blue and red diamonds, into the dense pine-and-oak forest. The hardwoods of the forest in this section of the park are rather mature, and you won't be hard-pressed to find impressively large trees growing by the trail. Follow the trail uphill and continue on the path for 400 feet until you reach a split in the trail. Stay to the right (north) and follow the trail into the forest. The path is very well marked and maintained. The trail signs are borderline overkill, as you will find them almost every 50 feet. Yet I have become lost on a trail before, and so I can very much appreciate the presence of anything that will keep me from straying from the path.

Over the next 0.7 mile the trail traverses a series of small hills as it heads toward the shore of Jordan Lake. The lake comes into view right before the trail steeply descends closer toward the edge of the lake, where the trail splits. To the right (north), a spur trail leads to an overlook with impressive views of the lake. Stay left (southwest) and continue on the Blue Trail for 1.4 miles. The trail curves around to the left and begins heading on a southwest bearing. The path descends a hill to a gravel road. Cross the gravel road and continue hiking along the Blue Trail, with the shore of Jordan Lake to your right, until you reach a junction. To the right (south), the Red Trail leads downhill toward a section of the New Hope Overlook area of the park called Area B. Stay straight (southeast) and continue uphill toward the Blue Trailhead.

After just 450 feet you come to another junction with the Red Trail. To the right (south), the Red Trail leads toward Area B. Stay to the left (northeast) and continue on the Blue Trail. The next section of the trail is marked with red and blue diamonds, and from here it is only 0.5 mile back to the trailhead, but this is the hardest part of the hike. The forest becomes thicker, and the trail climbs steeply uphill. Over the first 0.2 mile of this section, the trail climbs 198 feet in elevation, only to descend 219 feet to the trailhead over the next 0.2 mile, crossing a gravel road on the way down and reaching the trailhead and parking lot.

Nearby Attractions

More than 22 miles of hiking trails are spread out around Jordan Lake Recreation Area at the Ebenezer Church (see page 175), New Hope Overlook, Vista Point, Seaforth (see page 180), Parker's Creek, Crosswinds Campground, and Poplar Point Campground Recreation Areas.

Swift Creek Bluffs Nature Preserve (see page 111) is 16 miles to the east of Jordan Lake. A 1.2-mile trail follows along Swift Creek and leads to a small clearing with views of the creek and the towering bluffs along the creek bank.

Fourteen miles to the east is Fred G. Bond Metro Park (see pages 50 and 55), a 310-acre park with more than 4 miles of walking and biking trails that center on Bond Lake. The park is also the intersection for several of Cary's greenway trails, including Black Creek Greenway, Oxford Hunt Greenway, and White Oak Greenway.

Hemlock Bluffs Nature Preserve (see page 66) has nearly 4 miles of hiking trails and is 15 miles to the east of Jordan Lake. The trails at Hemlock Bluffs traverse small hills and lead to steep bluffs with views of Swift Creek below. The park is designated to protect clusters of eastern hemlocks on the north-facing bluffs and features a nature center geared toward young children.

Directions

Jordan Lake State Recreation Area is 24 miles south of Durham, off US 64. From downtown Durham the drive to the park usually takes 35 minutes. Note that the park address does not work well with most GPS units.

From Durham, take I-40 West toward Chapel Hill and follow it 4.7 miles. Take the NC 751 exit, Exit 274, toward Jordan Lake. Turn left onto NC 751/Hope Valley Road and continue to follow NC 751 for 12.2 miles. Turn right onto US 64 West toward Wilsonville and follow it 3.8 miles. Turn left onto State Park Road and follow it 4.5 miles. Turn right on County Road 1906 and continue 2.3 miles, following the signs toward New Hope Overlook and the boat ramp. Turn right on County Road 1910, which leads to the New Hope Overlook boat ramp and parking lot.

26

Jordan Lake State Recreation Area:

Old Oak Trail

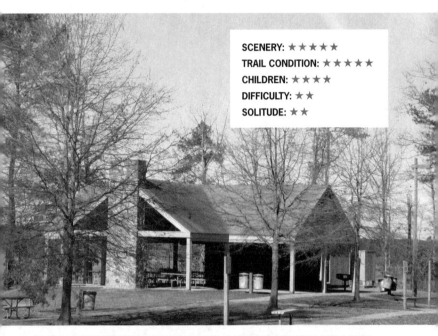

SCENERY: ★ ★ ★ ★
TRAIL CONDITION: ★ ★ ★ ★ ★
CHILDREN: ★ ★ ★ ★
DIFFICULTY: ★ ★
SOLITUDE: ★ ★

A LARGE PICNIC PAVILION ON JORDAN LAKE IS THE PERFECT SPOT FOR A REST WHERE YOU CAN TAKE IN THE SURROUNDING SCENERY OF THE LAKE.

GPS TRAILHEAD COORDINATES: N35° 42.489' W79° 01.479'

DISTANCE & CONFIGURATION: 1.6-mile balloon

HIKING TIME: 1 hour

HIGHLIGHTS: Jordan Lake, ponds, and historical farm sites

ELEVATION: 226' at trailhead to 266' at peak

ACCESS: May–August: Daily, 8 a.m.–9 p.m.; September–October and March–April: Daily, 8 a.m.–8 p.m.; November–February: Daily, 8 a.m.–6 p.m.; closed December 25. Memorial Day–Labor Day: daily, $6 admission; April–May and September on weekends and holidays: $6 admission; otherwise free.

MAPS: Online at ncparks.gov, at the park's visitor center, and at the trailhead kiosk

FACILITIES: Boat ramp, restrooms, water fountains, designated beaches, picnic pavilions, and playgrounds

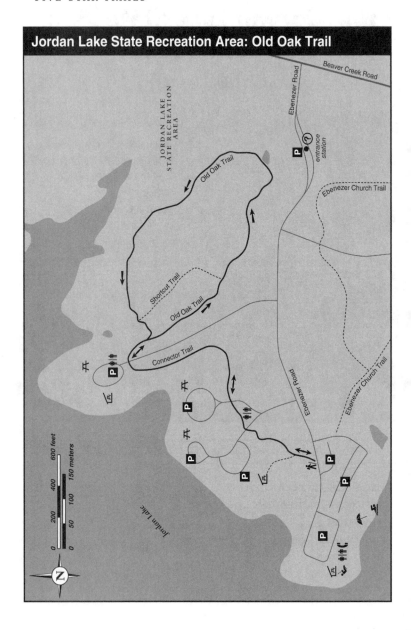

Jordan Lake State Recreation Area: Old Oak Trail

WHEELCHAIR ACCESS: No

COMMENTS: This park is very popular in the summer, when the boating crowd arrives to enjoy the 14,000 acres of water in the reservoir. The trails are heavily used on holidays and weekends, especially in the summer. The best time to enjoy the park is on weekdays during the spring and fall, which are also coincidentally the seasons in which the weather is best suited for hiking. Dogs are welcome on the trails as long as they are well behaved and kept on leashes no longer than 6 feet.

CONTACTS: 919-362-0586; ncparks.gov

Overview

There are two trails in the Ebenezer Church Recreation Area, the Ebenezer Church Trail and the Old Oak Trail. This route follows the Old Oak Trail, an easy 1-mile loop that begins at the Ebenezer Picnic Area A and passes two ponds as well as historic farm sites. The short-cut trail reduces the length of the trail to 0.5 mile, making this route exceptional for young children. The nearby Ebenezer Church Trail, also an easy 1-mile loop, explores the site of the historic Ebenezer Church and passes by a large pond. The Ebenezer Church Recreation Area has designated beaches and several picnic pavilions, so it is easy to spend a full day in the area.

Route Details

Park your vehicle at the lot on the far western side of the Ebenezer Church Recreation Area. Cross the road north of the parking lot, or the opposite direction of the lake, at the crosswalk to reach the Connector Trailhead. The trail is marked with red diamonds and descends for 150 feet to a split in the trail. To the left (northwest), the trail leads to picnic shelter two. Stay to the right (northeast), toward the Old Oak Trailhead. The trail continues through a dense forest and crosses a road that leads to a parking lot. You pass a restroom with water fountains on your right and can see views of the lake through the forest to your left.

The trail crosses the paved road and passes a picnic area on your left before descending to the lake's edge. Continue for 0.3 mile to the parking lot, with a large picnic pavilion on the edge of the lake. The trail continues at the Old Oak Trailhead, which is marked with a kiosk at the southeastern side of the parking lot. The path descends 200 feet to a split in the trail. For this route stay straight (southeast) and continue on the Old Oak Trail.

After 350 feet you reach a split in the trail. To the left is the Shortcut Trail. If you want to cut the trail short and make it a 0.5-mile hike, then you can take this Shortcut Trail to the other side of the Old Oak Trail, turn left, and follow the Old Oak Trail back to the Connector Trail, which you can then follow back to the parking lot where you started. To continue on the Old Oak Trail, stay straight (southeast). The Old Oak Trail traverses a beautiful and predominately pine forest for 0.1 mile until you reach an interpretive kiosk marking a small pond. The trail descends gradually from here for 0.2 mile, and then climbs gently uphill for another 0.1 mile until you reach a split in the trail. The other side of the Shortcut Trail splits to the left (southeast) uphill. This wouldn't be any shortcut at all at this point, so stay straight (west) and continue on the Old Oak Trail.

From here, follow the Old Oak Trail for 0.1 mile back to the Old Oak Trailhead, at the parking lot with the large picnic pavilion on the edge of Jordan Lake. Cross the parking lot and follow the trail on which you came in; the trail here is marked with a sign that simply reads TRAIL TO BEACH. At this point, backtrack on the Connector Trail and continue 0.4 mile to the parking lot where you started.

Nearby Attractions

More than 22 miles of hiking trails are spread out around Jordan Lake Recreation Area at the Ebenezer Church, New Hope Overlook (see page 169), Vista Point, Seaforth (see page 180), Parker's Creek, Crosswinds Campground, and Poplar Point Campground Recreation Areas.

Swift Creek Bluffs Nature Preserve (see page 111) is 16 miles to the east of Jordan Lake. A 1.2-mile trail follows along Swift Creek and leads to a small clearing with views of the creek and the towering bluffs along the creek bank.

Fourteen miles to the east is Fred G. Bond Metro Park (see pages 50 and 55), a 310-acre park with more than 4 miles of walking and biking trails that center on Bond Lake. The park is also the intersection for several of Cary's greenway trails, including Black Creek Greenway, Oxford Hunt Greenway, and White Oak Greenway.

Hemlock Bluffs Nature Preserve (see page 66) has nearly 4 miles of hiking trails and is 15 miles to the east of Jordan Lake. The trails at Hemlock Bluffs traverse small hills and lead to steep bluffs with views of Swift Creek below. The park is designated to protect clusters of eastern hemlocks on the north-facing bluffs and features a nature center geared toward young children.

Directions

Jordan Lake State Recreation Area is 24 miles south of Durham, off US 64. From downtown Durham the drive to the park usually takes 35 minutes. Note that the park address does not work well with most GPS units.

From Durham, take I-40 West toward Chapel Hill and follow it 4.7 miles. Take the NC 751 exit, Exit 274, toward Jordan Lake. Turn left onto NC 751/Hope Valley Road and continue to follow NC 751 for 12.2 miles. Turn right onto US 64 West toward Wilsonville and follow it 3.8 miles. Turn left onto State Park Road and follow it 2.3 miles. Turn right onto Ebenezer Church Road and follow the road to the parking lot, at the western tip of the recreation area.

27

Jordan Lake State Recreation Area:
Seaforth Pond Trail

SCENERY: ★ ★ ★ ★ ★
TRAIL CONDITION: ★ ★ ★ ★ ★
CHILDREN: ★ ★ ★ ★ ★
DIFFICULTY: ★ ★
SOLITUDE: ★ ★

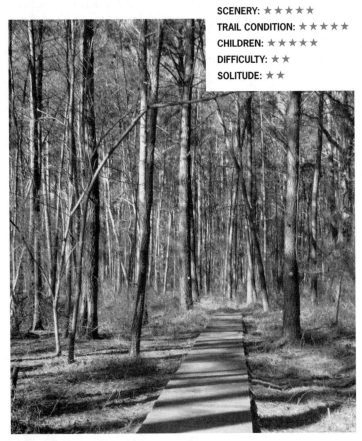

BOARDWALKS THROUGH BOGGY SECTIONS KEEP YOUR FEET DRY ALONG THE SEAFORTH POND TRAIL.

GPS TRAILHEAD COORDINATES: N35° 43.561' W79° 02.108'
DISTANCE & CONFIGURATION: 1.4-mile loop
HIKING TIME: 1 hour
HIGHLIGHTS: Jordan Lake, swimming beach, ponds, and wetland boardwalks

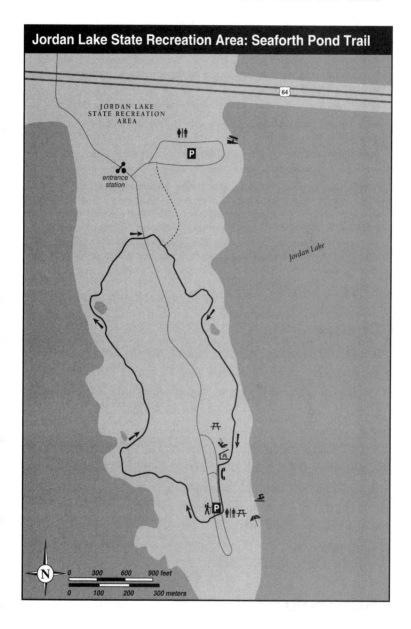

ELEVATION: 228' at trailhead to 235' at peak and 215' at lowest point

ACCESS: May–August: Daily, 8 a.m.–9 p.m.; September–October and March–April: Daily, 8 a.m.–8 p.m.; November–February: Daily, 8 a.m.–6 p.m.; closed December 25. Memorial Day–Labor Day: daily, $6 admission; April–May and September on weekends and holidays: $6 admission; otherwise, free.

MAPS: Online at ncparks.gov, at the park's visitor center, and at the trailhead kiosk

FACILITIES: Boat ramp, restrooms, showers, water fountains, designated beaches, picnic pavilions, and playground

WHEELCHAIR ACCESS: None on the trail. However, the beaches, restrooms, picnic facilities, and playground are all wheelchair-accessible.

COMMENTS: This park is very popular in the summer, when the boating and swimming crowd arrives to enjoy the 14,000 acres of water in the reservoir and the designated swimming beach at Seaforth. The trails are heavily used on holidays and weekends, especially in the summer. The best time to enjoy the park is on weekdays during the spring and fall, which are also coincidentally the seasons in which the weather is best suited for hiking. Dogs are welcome on the trails as long as they are well behaved and kept on leashes no longer than 6 feet.

CONTACTS: 919-362-0586; ncparks.gov

Overview

The Seaforth Recreation Area is centrally located in Jordan Lake State Recreation Area, right off US 64 west of Wilsonville. The Pond Trail is nearly a complete loop. It begins on the western side of the Seaforth parking lot and traverses a mixed pine-and-hardwood forest. Boardwalks along the way keep your hiking shoes from trudging through the wetland portions of the trail, where you will find buttonbush, black needlerush, and other wetland plants. Along the way, the path offers enjoyable views of Jordan Lake and passes by three small ponds. The trail circles back around to the parking lot and ends at picnic pavilion nine, a large, covered shelter on the edge of Jordan Lake to the north of the designated swimming beach. Bring your swimsuit and enjoy a day at Seaforth after hiking the Pond Trail.

Route Details

Park your vehicle at the Seaforth Beach parking lot. This is a very large parking lot that can accommodate the large crowds that come to enjoy the popular Seaforth Beach in the warmer months. The Seaforth Recreation Area, including the boat ramp and the trail, is one of the few areas in Jordan Lake State Recreation Area that is open year-round. If you want to explore other areas of the park, call ahead, as the trails are fairly spread out; you wouldn't want to drive all the way to a hiking area in the park to find it closed during the winter.

This hike is great for children. Apart from the fact that the trail is nice and level and considerably short, there is a playground, swimming beach, plenty of picnic shelters and pavilions, and even a sand volleyball court at Seaforth. One thing to keep in mind is that after exceptionally heavy rainfalls in this area, the western section of the trail can become flooded, leaving parts of the trail under water. The park has built several boardwalks to accommodate hikers, but there are still sections that can be left under water, and even days after a hard rain, these sections can be pretty muddy. These areas become submerged because they are low-lying wetlands; when they are dry, this part of the trail offers a very interesting ecosystem to explore, with water-loving plants that are only found in these types of wetland habitats. The Seaforth Pond Trail is also a great trail for runners. The path's short length makes it compatible with trail runners who want to run the loop several times and never stray too far from the parking lot.

The kiosk and trailhead are at the west side of the parking lot, directly across from the swimming beach. The trail, marked with red diamonds, follows the lakeshore and crosses several raised boardwalks over the first 0.3 mile until you reach the first of three small ponds. In another 0.3 mile you will reach the second pond on the right side of the trail.

Along this section of the trail you reach several clearings along the shore of the lake to the left of the trail. These can be great spots for a picnic or for watching the many species of birds that inhabit the forest surrounding Jordan Lake. The most famous and recognizable of the feathered friends that inhabit the area is the bald eagle. Jordan Lake State Recreation Area is one of the largest summertime homes of the bald eagle, and the population has increased dramatically since the flooding of the reservoir in 1983. The bald eagle is still protected, and interpretive programs about the birds are conducted throughout the year at Jordan Lake.

Ascend the wooden steps and follow along the raised berm on the edge of the pond. After passing the pond the trail curves around to the right (east) and becomes considerably wider. Here on the left is a narrow meadow surrounded by young pine trees.

Continue on the Seaforth Pond Trail for 0.2 mile and then cross the paved road. Continue for 250 feet until you reach a split in the trail. To the left (north) a spur trail leads to the boat ramp, but continue straight (east) toward the shore of Jordan Lake. From here the trail descends to rejoin the lakeshore, passing the third small pond on the left before climbing up to picnic pavilion nine. Here you reach a picnic area, the eastern side of the parking lot, and the end of the trail.

Nearby Attractions

More than 22 miles of hiking trails are spread out around Jordan Lake Recreation Area at the Ebenezer Church (see page 175), New Hope Overlook (see page 169), Vista Point, Seaforth, Parker's Creek, Crosswinds Campground, and Poplar Point Campground Recreation Areas.

Swift Creek Bluffs Nature Preserve (see page 111) is 16 miles to the east of Jordan Lake. A 1.2-mile trail follows along Swift Creek and leads to a small clearing with views of the creek and the towering bluffs along the creek bank.

Fourteen miles to the east is Fred G. Bond Metro Park (see pages 50 and 55), a 310-acre park with more than 4 miles of walking and biking trails that center on Bond Lake. The park is also the intersection for several of Cary's greenway trails, including Black Creek Greenway, Oxford Hunt Greenway, and White Oak Greenway.

Hemlock Bluffs Nature Preserve (see page 66) has nearly 4 miles of hiking trails and is 15 miles to the east of Jordan Lake. The trails at Hemlock Bluffs traverse small hills and lead to steep bluffs with views of Swift Creek below. The park is designated to protect clusters of eastern hemlocks on the north-facing bluffs and features a nature center geared toward young children.

Directions

Jordan Lake State Recreation Area is 24 miles south of Durham, off US 64. From downtown Durham the drive to the park usually takes 35 minutes. Note that the park address does not work well with most GPS units.

From Durham, take I-40 West toward Chapel Hill and follow it 4.7 miles. Take the NC 751 exit, Exit 274, toward Jordan Lake. Turn left onto NC 751/Hope Valley Road and continue to follow NC 751 for 12.2 miles. Turn right onto US 64 West toward Wilsonville and follow it 5.8 miles. Seaforth Recreation Area will be on the left (south) side of US 64.

28

North Carolina Botanical Garden

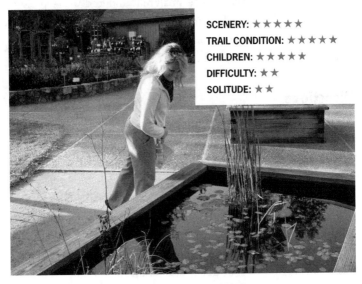

SCENERY: ★ ★ ★ ★ ★
TRAIL CONDITION: ★ ★ ★ ★ ★
CHILDREN: ★ ★ ★ ★ ★
DIFFICULTY: ★ ★
SOLITUDE: ★ ★

CHECK OUT THE FISH PONDS AT THE END OF THE TRAIL.

GPS TRAILHEAD COORDINATES: N35° 53.991' W79° 01.956'

DISTANCE & CONFIGURATION: 0.5-mile loop

HIKING TIME: 1 hour

HIGHLIGHTS: Botanical gardens and Education Center

ELEVATION: Negligible—295' at trailhead to 301' at peak

ACCESS: Day after Labor Day–day before Memorial Day: Monday–Friday, 8 a.m.–5 p.m.; Saturday, 9 a.m.–5 p.m.; Sunday, 1–5 p.m. Memorial Day–Labor Day: Monday–Friday, 8 a.m.–5 p.m.; Saturday, 9 a.m.–6 p.m.; Sunday, 1–6 p.m. Closed Martin Luther King Jr. Day, Thanksgiving, and a week during winter holidays. Free.

MAPS: At the Education Center and trailhead kiosk

FACILITIES: Restrooms, water fountains, education center, and picnic area

WHEELCHAIR ACCESS: Yes

COMMENTS: While the garden hosts a diverse collection of plants that bloom throughout the year, the best times to visit the garden are during the spring, when more plants are blossoming, and during the fall, when the trees are at the peak of their colorful display. Leashed dogs are allowed on the Piedmont Nature Trails but not in the gardens or around or in the education center.

CONTACTS: 919-962-0522; ncbg.unc.edu

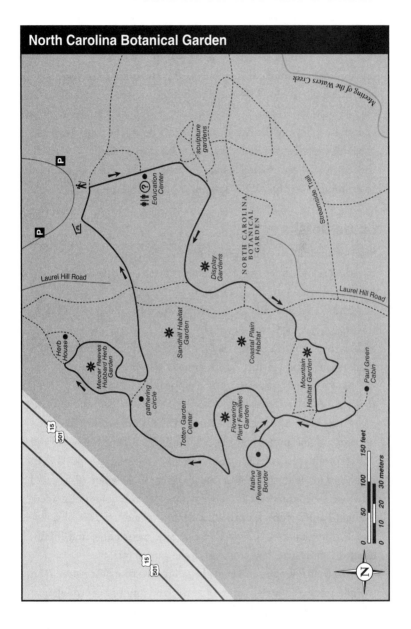

North Carolina Botanical Garden

Overview

The North Carolina Botanical Garden, administered by the University of North Carolina at Chapel Hill, is 5 miles southeast of downtown Chapel Hill. In 1744 the first European settler in Chapel Hill chose this location for his homesite, and today you can explore the garden by following the paved paths throughout. The route begins at the Education Center and follows the main path. From here, you walk through 14 collections and display gardens and have the opportunity to examine more than 2,100 species of plants and trees.

Route Details

Start in front of the education center. Walk straight (south) on the paved path and under the arbor that connects the gift shop with the Mouzon Classroom. The education center houses classrooms, an auditorium, seminar rooms, an exhibit hall, a botanical art and illustration gallery, the Green Gardener Reference Room, and a gift shop. Follow the path into the display gardens and the sculpture displays. Each fall, the garden installs its annual "Sculpture in the Garden" exhibition, displaying a variety of sculptures throughout the gardens that visitors can purchase.

This garden really began when William Chambers Coker, the university's first professor of botany, and his student Henry Roland Totten proposed a botanical garden south of the main campus. Plantings were made in the 1940s, but it was in 1952 when 70 forested acres were dedicated for the development of the botanical garden. William Lanier Hunt, a horticulturist and former student of Coker and Totten, donated 103 acres of dramatic creek gorge and rhododendron bluffs, which were added to the garden facility.

In the 1960s the university began conducting field research on the adjoining 367-acre tract of old farmland and native woodlands, which was formally dedicated in 1984 as the Mason Farm Biological Reserve. The reserve provides research facilities for ecology, bird behavior, population biology, genetics, and developmental biology projects. In 2000 the Education Center, designated a Platinum building under the Leadership in Energy and Environmental Design rating system of the U.S. Green Building Council, was launched.

Circle the gardens and follow the trail to the Coastal Plains Habitat Garden. The Coastal Plains Garden and Sandhills Habitat Garden to the north represent the wide range of ecosystems present in the eastern part of the state. In the outer coastal plain you find myrtles and carnivorous plants, such as Venus flytraps and pitcher plants. This garden is annually burned to simulate the processes that are part of the endangered longleaf-pine ecosystem, where fire plays an important role in promoting the growth of a high diversity of plants.

Walk 300 feet until the trail splits. Turn left (southwest) and follow the path around to the west, passing another display garden with whimsical sculpture. Here you pass a fence and then reach another intersection. After 250 feet turn left (south) into the Mountain Habitat Garden. The Mountain Habitat Garden has plants and trees on display that are characteristic of the mountainous areas of the southern Appalachians at elevations ranging from 1,500 feet to 6,684 feet. Here you will find many plants native to the western boundary of North Carolina, including wildflowers that bloom in the spring, such as trilliums, bluebells, bloodroots, liverleafs, and Oconee bells. You will also see mountain laurels, azaleas, rhododendrons, Canadian hemlocks, white pines, tulip trees, and many species of ferns.

Follow the trail for 200 feet until you reach a four-way intersection. Turn left (south) toward the historic Paul Green Cabin, where its namesake, a playwright, created many of his works. The trail passes through the cabin and circles around to the north and to the native perennial border, a collection of native perennials, shrubs, and small trees designed to bloom throughout the growing season and to supply nectar for pollinators from spring to fall.

Follow the trail as it circles a large sculpture and then veers to the left toward the area housing the aquatic and carnivorous plants. All of the aquatic plants in the water gardens are native to the southeastern United States. The collection includes American white water lilies, American lotus lilies, and heartleaf pickerelweed. You can also spot bullfrog tadpoles, goldfish, and koi that live in the ponds. The carnivorous-plant collection, known as one of the best in the Southeast, displays numerous species of pitcher plants, sundews, butterworts, and Venus flytraps.

An arbor 50 feet from the Native Perennial Border marks the entrance to the Flowering Plant Families' Garden. Turn right (north) and follow alongside Totten Garden Center and toward the giant chessboard. The trail splits and either way leads to the gathering circle, a mosaic stone–tiled area.

The Totten Garden Center, to the south of the gathering circle, now serves as the hub of horticultural and propagation activities. The landscaped garden areas around the Totten Garden Center feature native Southeastern plants. The center is also used for a testing ground, where drought-tolerant plants, ferns that do well in sunny locations, evergreen ground covers, and flowering perennials are displayed. From the gathering circle, continue north for 250 feet to the herb garden and follow the trail to the right (east) to the Herb House. From the Herb House, follow the trail back around to the gathering circle. Turn left at the gathering circle and continue for 300 feet, passing the cattail gate and returning to the parking lot and trailhead.

Nearby Attractions

Chapel Hill and the University of North Carolina at Chapel Hill campus are 5 miles northwest of the botanical garden. Downtown Chapel Hill (see page 132) is integrated into the campus, and you can explore the campus and the nearby charming business district along Franklin Street. There are plenty of restaurants, cafés, and shopping opportunities here. If you're going to be staying in the downtown Chapel Hill area overnight, the Carolina Inn, at 211 Pittman St., is a charming and highly recommended accommodation. It is listed on the National

Register of Historic Places and is a member of the National Trust's Historic Hotels of America.

Fifteen miles to the south is Jordan Lake State Recreation Area, with more than 22 miles of hiking trails spread out around Jordan Lake at the Ebenezer Church (see page 175), New Hope Overlook (see page 169), Vista Point, Seaforth (see page 180), Parker's Creek, Crosswinds Campground, and Poplar Point Campground Recreation Areas.

Seventeen miles east of the botanical garden you can visit the William B. Umstead State Park (see pages 117 and 123). This 5,579-acre park offers more than 20 miles of hiking trails, as well as opportunities for paddling and boating on Big Lake, and biking and horseback riding on the bridle and biking trails throughout the park. Umstead also has tent and trailer camping for $20 per day. Showers, water, and restrooms are available in the campgrounds.

Directions

From Raleigh, take I-40 West and follow it 16 miles. Merge onto NC 54 West via Exit 273A toward Chapel Hill and follow it 3.1 miles. Merge onto US 15 South toward Carrboro/Pittsboro and follow it 0.8 mile. Turn left onto Old Mason Farm Road and follow it 0.1 mile. On the right you will see 100 Old Mason Road and the North Carolina Botanical Garden.

From Durham, take Durham Chapel Hill Boulevard and follow it for 5.2 miles. Durham Chapel Hill Boulevard becomes US 15 South; follow it 3.8 miles. Turn left onto Old Mason Farm Road and follow it 0.1 mile. On the right you will see 100 Old Mason Road and the North Carolina Botanical Garden.

Occoneechee Mountain Loop Trail

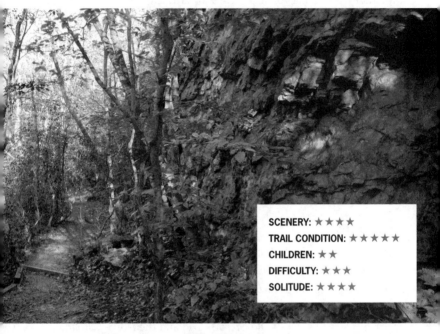

YOU WILL FIND INTERESTING ROCK FORMATIONS SUCH AS THIS ONE ALONG THE OCCONEECHEE MOUNTAIN LOOP TRAIL.

GPS TRAILHEAD COORDINATES: N36° 03.636' W79° 07.059'

DISTANCE & CONFIGURATION: 2.3-mile loop

HIKING TIME: 1.5 hours

HIGHLIGHTS: Occoneechee Mountain summit, rock formations, ponds, and bluffs

ELEVATION: 654' at trailhead to 754' at peak and 507' at lowest point

ACCESS: November–February: Daily, 8 a.m.–6 p.m. March–April and September–October: Daily, 8 a.m.–8 p.m. May–August: Daily, 8 a.m.–9 p.m.; closed December 25. Free.

MAPS: Online at ncparks.gov, at the Eno River State Park office, and at the trailhead kiosk

FACILITIES: Restrooms

WHEELCHAIR ACCESS: No

COMMENTS: The Occoneechee Mountain State Natural Area is serviced by Eno River State Park. The physical addresses for these two parks are the same, and if you put the address for the park into a GPS unit, it will lead you to the Eno River State Park office. The best way to find the park is to put the GPS trailhead coordinates (see previous page) into your GPS unit or follow the directions on page 197. The park welcomes dogs as long as they are on a leash no longer than 6 feet.

CONTACTS: 919-383-1686; ncparks.gov

Overview

The 190-acre Occoneechee Mountain State Natural Area is 10 miles northwest of Durham and offers more than 4 miles of hiking trails. The main trail in the park is the Occoneechee Mountain Loop Trail. This route goes around the base of the mountain and passes the spur Summit Trail, which leads to the summit of Occoneechee Mountain, the highest point in Orange County and the site of one of the most important natural areas in the Triangle. This spur leaves the steep climb to the summit as an option, but it is highly recommended and offers spectacular views of the surrounding rolling landscape.

The trail starts from the parking lot at the end of Virginia Cates Road, next to two small fishing ponds. The path leads around the base of the mountain, climbing several hills and traversing a rich diversity of forest habitat before returning to the parking lot.

Route Details

Follow the gravel Virginia Cates Road past the fishing ponds to the parking area near the Occoneechee Mountain Loop Trailhead, behind the restrooms on the left (west) side of the parking lot. Follow the 4-foot-wide unpaved path to the west; over the next 1.3 miles you will climb uphill and then head back down toward the Eno River. The trail follows the river's edge and then begins climbing again, this time ascending a set of wooden steps. At the top of the steps, on the right side of the trail, you reach a very interesting sheer rock wall that has been cut away by the Eno River, to your left.

While hiking in the park you might encounter deer, ground-hogs, and wild turkey that feed on the acorns and berries produced

Occoneechee Mountain Loop Trail

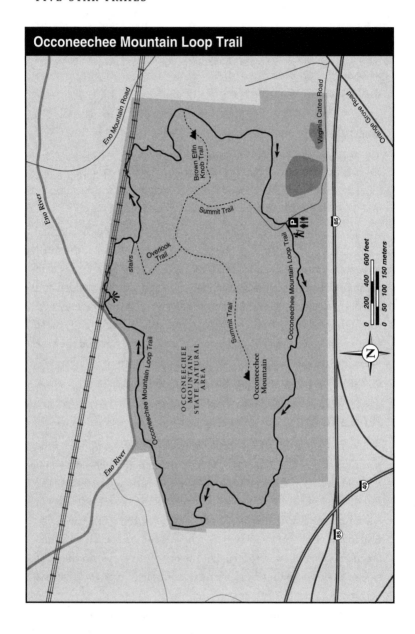

by the chestnut oaks and other plants found in the park. The Occoneechee Mountain summit is 867 feet high, and the relatively undisturbed forest on the summit includes a stand of chestnut trees that is considered one of the best stands in the region. One of the rarest animal species found in the park is the brown elfin butterfly. This species of butterfly is believed to have survived in the Occoneechee area since the ice age; the nearest population of brown elfin butterflies is nearly 100 miles away, in the Appalachian Mountains of western North Carolina.

The trail curves around to the right (north) and climbs a very steep hill, gaining 214 feet of elevation in just 470 feet, to a trail junction. From here the climb seems worth it, and you have a great view of the northern slope of Occoneechee Mountain, its north face a cliff of sheer rock. It is quite an impressive view. To the right (south) a spur trail leads to an overlook with better views of the rock cliff wall of Occoneechee Mountain. Stay to the left (east) and continue hiking on the Occoneechee Mountain Loop Trail.

The land around Occoneechee Mountain was originally inhabited by the Occonechi band of American Indians. It is believed that

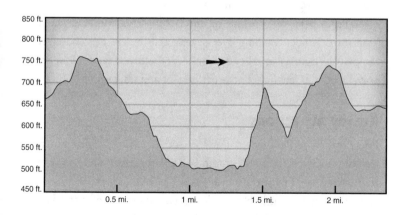

these early Americans traveled to this region from the west due to the types of artifacts and designs in their pottery that they left behind. Europeans settled in the area during the Colonial period, and a textile mill and the surrounding village occupied this site along the Eno River until 1956. The first land purchase by the North Carolina Division of Parks and Recreation was made in 1997, and now the park has grown to more than 190 acres.

Continue 0.2 mile, following the trail as it curves around to the right (south) and then climbs up a set of wooden stairs to the intersection with the Overlook Trail. To the right (west) the Overlook Trail climbs up to an intersection with the Summit Trail, which leads uphill to the summit of Occoneechee Mountain. From here it's about a mile to the summit and back. It's up to you if you want to extend the hike, but I highly recommend doing so—the views from the top are great. To keep the trail a loop around the base of the mountain, stay to the left (east) and continue hiking on the Occoneechee Mountain Loop Trail.

After 0.4 mile you reach a trail junction. To the right (west), the Brown Elfin Knob Trail connects to the Summit Trail and leads to the summit of Occoneechee Mountain. Stay straight and continue on the Occoneechee Mountain Trail toward the parking lot.

From here you continue on the Occoneechee Mountain Loop Trail for 0.3 mile, climbing over several hills before descending to the gravel Virginia Cates Road. Turn left (southwest) and follow the gravel road 200 feet back to the parking lot and trailhead.

Nearby Attractions

Eno River State Park (see pages 151 and 157) is 10 miles northeast of the Occoneechee Mountain State Natural Area and has more than 24 miles of hiking trails to explore. One of the most scenic areas along the Eno River is Bobbitt Hole, which can be reached by walking the 1.7-mile Bobbitt Hole Loop Trail (see page 151).

Fourteen miles east of Occoneechee Mountain is West Point on the Eno (see page 204), a 388-acre Durham city park with more than 3 miles of hiking trails that further explore the Eno River and the surrounding forest. Within the park, take a tour of a replica of the original West Point Mill and buy some fresh stone-ground flour and cornmeal, which are made on-site. Swimming and fishing are very popular in the park as well.

Directions

From Durham, take I-85 South to Exit 164 toward Hillsborough. Turn right onto South Churton Street and follow it 0.1 mile. Take the second left onto Mayo Street and follow it 0.3 mile. Turn left onto Orange Grove Road and follow it 0.2 mile. Take the second right onto Virginia Cates Road and follow it 0.3 mile before entering the park. If you reach Patriots Pointe Drive, you've gone about 0.3 mile too far.

30

Sarah P. Duke Gardens

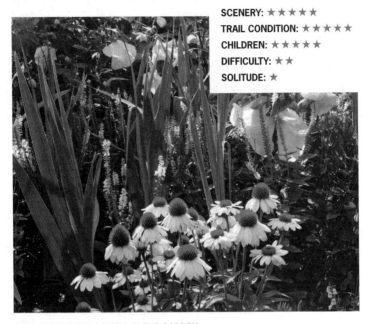

SCENERY: ★ ★ ★ ★
TRAIL CONDITION: ★ ★ ★ ★ ★
CHILDREN: ★ ★ ★ ★ ★
DIFFICULTY: ★ ★
SOLITUDE: ★

CONEFLOWERS BLOOMING IN THE GARDEN

GPS TRAILHEAD COORDINATES: N36° 00.105' W78° 55.929'

DISTANCE & CONFIGURATION: 1.1-mile loop

HIKING TIME: 1 hour

HIGHLIGHTS: Doris Duke Center and Gardens, H. L. Blomquist Garden, Historic Gardens, and W. L. Culberson Asiatic Arboretum

ELEVATION: 390' at trailhead to 339' at lowest point

ACCESS: Daily, 8 a.m.–sunset; free

MAPS: Online at www.hr.duke.edu/dukegardens and at the garden's visitor center

FACILITIES: Restrooms, water fountains, and café

WHEELCHAIR ACCESS: Many of the trails are accessible by wheelchair. However, there are some steps and gravel trails that can be difficult to navigate with a wheelchair. The staff at the visitor center are happy to assist those with disabilities in determining which trails are recommended.

COMMENTS: This is a very popular attraction. Be prepared for crowds.

CONTACTS: 919-684-3698; www.hr.duke.edu/dukegardens

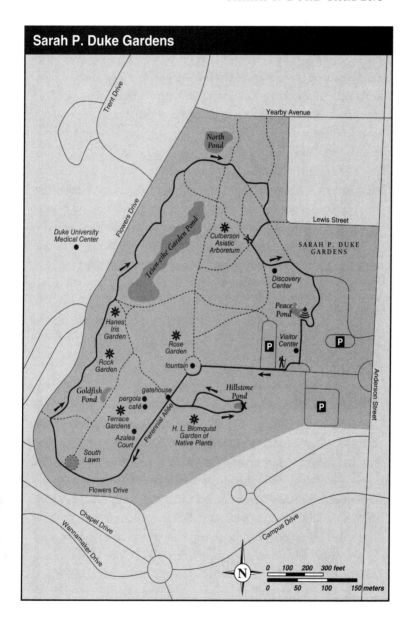

Sarah P. Duke Gardens

Overview

Considered the crown jewel of Duke University, the 55-acre Sarah P. Duke Gardens is a not-to-be-missed, artfully designed and sculpted landscape. One of the premier gardens in the United States, it hosts more than 300,000 visitors a year. If you can visit only a few places while you are in the Raleigh/Durham area, I highly recommend that you take the time to explore this impressive garden.

The Sarah P. Duke Gardens consists of four major parts. The Terrace Gardens, in the southwest section of the garden, are also called the Historic Gardens and contain the fish ponds, rose garden, and beautiful wisteria-covered terraces. The South Lawn, in the Terraces, was the location of the original garden. The H. L. Blomquist Garden of Native Plants, in the southeastern part of the garden, is a stunning representation of the flora of the southeastern United States. The William L. Culberson Asiatic Arboretum, in the northwest section, is devoted to plants of eastern Asia. In the eastern section of the garden you find the Doris Duke Center Gardens. Combined, the gardens offer 5 miles of allées, walks, and pathways.

Route Details

The university originally wanted to turn this valley land into a lake. There was a grand vision of luxurious fountains and a massive lake, but the plan was scrapped when the funding never materialized. The idea to build a garden at this site was proposed in the early 1930s by Dr. Frederic M. Hanes, an early member of the faculty of Duke Medical School. The doctor was taking daily strolls along a path through a debris-filled ravine when he thought about transforming the land into a garden filled with irises, his favorite flower. After a rather sizable $20,000 donation from Sarah P. Duke, a garden of 40,000 irises, 25,000 daffodils, 10,000 small bulbs, and many assorted annuals was constructed where the South Lawn stands today. Unfortunately, the designers did not take into account the fact that this ravine was at too low of an elevation for a proper and sustainable garden.

By 1936, just one year later, the entire garden was destroyed by flooding and heavy rains. The new garden, which you can experience today, was built as a memorial to Sarah P. Duke by her daughter, Mary Duke Biddle. High ground was smartly chosen as the planting site by Ellen Shipman, the pioneer landscape designer and architect. Of the more than 650 gardens Shipman designed, Sarah P. Duke Gardens is said to be her masterpiece and legacy.

There is so much to explore in these gardens, and while this route may only explore a portion of the trails, the path touches on the highlights. Feel free, of course, to explore these gardens on your own. Let this book simply be a guide and not the definitive route.

Start your trip from the garden entrance, north of the visitor center. Large stone columns and masterfully constructed iron Gothic-themed gates mark the entrance to the gardens. Follow the gravel path west for 350 feet until you reach the impressive round fountain. Surrounding the fountain is the fragrant Rose Garden. Follow the path around the fountain to the left (southwest) and continue for about 260 feet, passing a perennial flower garden called Perennial Allée. Turn left (east) into the Blomquist Garden and walk 90 feet, passing the gatehouse and information kiosk. You will reach a junction in the trail.

There are many spur trails in this garden. However, stay straight, walking through the Woodland Bridge Garden for 300 feet until you reach Hillstone Pond at the far eastern end of the trail. From here you can follow the path as it loops back around to the west and returns to the main trail, where you entered the Blomquist Garden at the gatehouse and kiosk. Once you reach the junction with the main trail, turn left (northwest) and head toward the South Lawn. During this section of the trail you will pass Azalea Court and the Pergola on your right. After 450 feet the trail curves to the right and starts heading toward the west. Shortly after the trail curves, you reach the South Lawn on your right, a large, open, grassy lawn where you are likely to find visitors picnicking, sunning, and playing Frisbee or holding an informal soccer game. It is a lively area of the garden and a great spot for people-watching.

Follow the trail 0.1 mile around the edge of the South Lawn until you arrive at a trail junction. A spur trail to the left heads toward Flowers Drive. Turn right (northeast). After 10 feet the trail splits. To the right, a short spur trail leads to an excellent view of the large Terrace Gardens. Stay to the left, continuing on the main path that borders Flowers Drive. After 400 feet you reach three spur trails on the right, one after the other. They all lead into the Rock Garden. Stay straight (north) and follow the main trail. After another 300 feet you reach a trail junction. This trail cuts through the garden, creating a path that separates the Historic Gardens from the Culberson Asiatic Arboretum. Stay straight on the main trail and head into the Asiatic Arboretum. Continue 0.2 mile, following alongside Flowers Drive and passing the very impressive daylily gardens, the Japanese Pavilion, and the Japanese Garden, one of my favorite sections. It is a very peaceful spot, and one that I encourage you to explore.

Immediately after the trail circles to the right (east), you reach a junction. To the left the trail leads to Yearby Avenue. To the right a trail cuts through the garden, heading south toward the round fountain. Stay straight and follow the trail toward the eastern edge of the Asiatic Arboretum.

After 200 feet you reach another junction. Stay to the left (east). After 100 feet you reach another spur trail to the left that leads to Yearby Avenue. Stay right (south) for 25 feet and then turn left at the split in the trail. After 50 more feet you will reach a four-way junction. Turn right (southwest) and follow the trail into the Doris Duke Center Gardens. After 200 feet you reach a trail junction. A breathtaking bridge is to your right. Turn left and walk 150 feet. At the split in the trail, keep left and pass the Discovery Center on your right. Walk 200 feet to a trail junction and turn right. After another 200 feet you will reach a junction with a service road that leads to the parking lot. Stay to the right and follow the path past lily-filled Peace Pond and back to the visitor center. The parking lot where you started is on the west side of the visitor center.

Nearby Attractions

A parcel of the 7,020-acre Duke Forest is adjacent to the Duke University campus (see page 144). Spread out over Alamance, Durham, and Orange Counties, the forest is broken up into six separate forest areas. You'll find more than 5 miles of hiking trails, including the popular 0.8-mile Shepherd Nature Trail off NC 751 at Gate C.

Downtown Durham (see page 139) is just 4 miles to the east of the Duke University campus. You can explore many of the highlights in the downtown district, including the Durham Bulls Athletic Park, Parrish Street financial district, and the American Tobacco and Warehouse Districts. Distinguished as one of the major hubs of tobacco distribution in the 1900s, as well as a financial capital for African Americans, downtown Durham today is experiencing a renaissance, with many of the spacious tobacco warehouses being transformed into lofty apartment buildings, restaurants, and shopping plazas. Experience the local flavor at Dame's Chicken & Waffles, or grab a hot dog and a box of Cracker Jacks and dig into a taste of Americana tradition with the Durham Bulls, America's most famous AAA baseball team.

Directions

From Raleigh, Sarah P. Duke Gardens is 25 miles to the northwest. Take Wade Avenue to I-40 West and follow I-40 for 9 miles. Merge onto NC 147 North via Exit 279B toward Durham/Downtown and follow it 9.7 miles. Take the Chapel Hill Street exit, Exit 13. Turn right onto West Chapel Hill Street and follow it 0.6 mile. West Chapel Hill Street becomes Duke University Road. Continue to follow Duke University Road 0.5 mile. Turn right onto Anderson Street and follow it 0.2 mile. The entrance to the garden will be on your left. If you reach Bynum Street, you've gone too far.

From Durham, take Duke University Road to Anderson Street. Turn right onto Anderson Street and follow it 0.2 mile. The entrance to the garden will be on your left. If you reach Bynum Street, you've gone too far.

31

West Point on the Eno:
Nature Trail

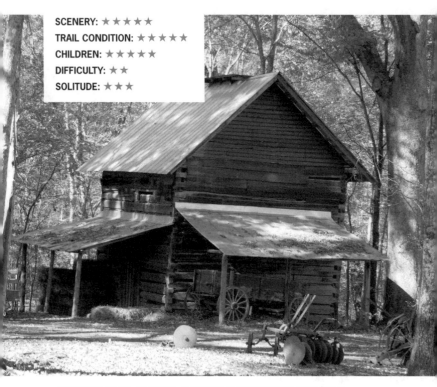

SCENERY: ★ ★ ★ ★
TRAIL CONDITION: ★ ★ ★ ★ ★
CHILDREN: ★ ★ ★ ★ ★
DIFFICULTY: ★ ★
SOLITUDE: ★ ★ ★

ALONG THE TRAIL YOU WILL DISCOVER HISTORIC FARM BUILDINGS.

GPS TRAILHEAD COORDINATES: N36° 04.123' W78° 54.516'

DISTANCE & CONFIGURATION: 0.7-mile balloon

HIKING TIME: 1 hour

HIGHLIGHTS: Mangum House, historic barn, Packhouse and Hugh Mangum Museum of Photography, and West Point Mill

ELEVATION: 335' at trailhead to 285' at lowest point

ACCESS: Trails: Daily, 8 a.m.–sunset. Historic buildings: Mid-March–mid-December: Saturday–Sunday, 1–5 p.m. Free.

MAPS: Online at enoriver.org and at the trailhead kiosk

FACILITIES: Restrooms, water fountains, and picnic facilities

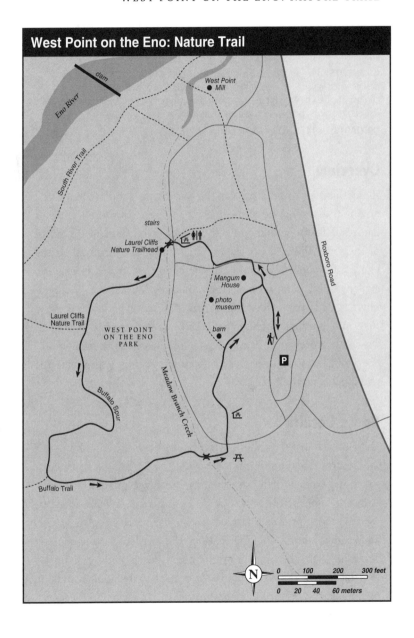

West Point on the Eno: Nature Trail

dam

Eno River

West Point
● Mill

South River Trail

stairs

Laurel Cliffs
Nature Trailhead ●

Mangum ●
House

● photo
museum

Laurel Cliffs
Nature Trail

WEST POINT
ON THE ENO
PARK

barn
●

Roxboro Road

P

Buffalo Spur

Meadow Branch Creek

Buffalo Trail

N

0   100   200   300 feet

0   20   40   60 meters

WHEELCHAIR ACCESS: The paths around the historic buildings are wheelchair-accessible. However, the nature trails behind the farmstead on the other side of the Eno River are unpaved and not accessible.

COMMENTS: There are several areas along the river to launch a canoe or kayak if you are interested in paddling some of the Eno. The park is popular with school groups and children. The best time to visit the park to avoid crowds is during the summer months, weekday mornings and evenings, and weekend mornings.

CONTACTS: 919-471-1623; enoriver.org

Overview

Along this trail you can explore the historic park and buildings that occupy the original homestead and mill-operation area. The park's landscape features rolling hills in the preserved lands to the north of the river. The trail is easy and only traverses a small hill at the end of the route. It begins near the historic Mangum House and explores the Packhouse and Hugh Mangum Museum of Photography, as well as the historic West Point Mill. The trail crosses the Eno River and meanders through the forest before curving back around to the south, crossing the Eno again, and leading to the western area of the park. Here the trail passes a historic barn before returning to the parking lot and trailhead.

Route Details

This 388-acre park, 6 miles north of downtown Durham, borders a 2-mile stretch of the scenic Eno River. Feel free to bring your canoe or kayak and experience the beauty of the Eno River. This area was originally the home of the Shocco and Eno American Indians. The first white settlers, primarily farmers and millers, arrived in the 1750s and established the West Point Mill at the excellent ford on the Eno River, accessible by roads from the north, south, and west. Thirty-two mills once dotted the Eno River, but due to the mill's ownership by notable and influential men, the growth of Durham to the south, and the mill's favorable location on the river, the West Point Mill was the most successful of them all.

The mill functioned from 1778 to 1942, and during that time it became a vital center for a community of around 300 families. There was a general store, blacksmith shop, cotton gin, sawmill, still, and post office. The name West Point—given to both the mill and the surrounding community—came from the fact that it was the most westerly point on the mail route from Raleigh to Roxboro. In 1942 the mill ceased operations when a flood resulting from a heavy rain broke the dam across the river. The building collapsed in 1973, but through the use of photographs of the original mill, the mill was reconstructed using materials from some of the other gristmills in the region. Today the West Point Mill grinds corn and wheat with power from the water of the Eno River, and the stone-ground meal and flour are sold in the mill's store.

Park your vehicle in the gravel parking lot. The trailhead and kiosk are at the north side of the parking lot. Follow the 5-foot-wide paved trail for 200 feet to the Mangum House on the left side of the trail. In the 1840s John Cabe McCown, a former owner of the West Point Mill, built this farmhouse as his residence. In 1891 the house was sold to Presley J. Mangum, who wanted to escape the growing town of Durham; the Mangum family lived in the house until 1968. The house was restored during this time, but it still features original mantels, woodwork, and rooms sided in original heart pine boards.

Walk past the house and continue on the trail for 80 feet until you reach the gravel road. Turn left (west) and walk 170 feet until you reach a break in the split rail fence. Turn right (west) and walk 200 feet through the meadow to the picnic area with restrooms; it looks more like a cabin. From here descend the paved steps and walk 125 feet to the gravel road and the Laurel Cliffs Nature Trailhead. Notice the rebuilt West Point Mill on the bank of the Eno River just to your right (east).

Cross the wooden bridge over the Meadow Branch Creek and continue on the unpaved nature trail that leads into the forest. It is well marked with white and yellow blazes and easy to follow. The trail curves around to the left (south), and after 0.1 mile it reaches a junction with the Laurel Cliffs Nature Trail, which leads to the river. Stay straight (south) and follow the trail 0.2 mile until you reach a split in the trail. The Buffalo Trail, to the right (west), also leads to the river. Stay to the left and continue back toward Meadow Creek. After 0.1 mile, you reach the Meadow Branch Creek again.

Turn left (east) and cross the wooden bridge over Meadow Branch Creek. Then cross the gravel road on the other side of the creek and walk toward the picnic pavilion, straight ahead. After 300 feet, and right before you reach the picnic pavilion, the trail veers to the left and enters a small forested area. Continue 225 feet until you reach the trail junction. Turn right (northeast), passing the historic barn on your left. The Hugh Mangum Museum of Photography will be straight ahead. The museum is located in one of the original buildings at West Point and was once used for handling tobacco. The museum hosts regular exhibits by many regional photographers, and it houses a permanent exhibit of Hugh Mangum's images and photography equipment.

Pass the photography museum and follow the path back to the Mangum House and the small garden behind the house. When you reach the circular trail in front of the garden, turn right (east) toward the front of the house. Here you rejoin the paved trail. Turn right (south) and follow the paved path back to the parking lot and trailhead.

Nearby Attractions

Eno River State Park (see pages 151 and 157) is 7 miles west of the West Point on the Eno, and it has more than 24 miles of hiking trails to explore. One of the most scenic areas along the Eno River is Bobbitt Hole, which can be reached by walking the 1.7-mile Bobbitt Hole Loop Trail (see page 151).

The 190-acre Occoneechee Mountain State Natural Area (see page 192), 7 miles west of West Point on the Eno, offers more than 4 miles of hiking trails.

Directions

From Raleigh, take I-40 West and follow it 9 miles. Merge onto NC 147 North via Exit 279B toward Durham/Downtown and follow it 5.7 miles. Take the Briggs Avenue exit, Exit 10, toward Durham Technical Community College and follow it 0.2 mile. Turn left onto South Briggs Avenue and follow it 0.2 mile. Merge onto NC 147 South via the ramp on the left and follow it 2.5 miles. Take the Ellis Road exit, Exit 8. Turn left onto Ellis Road and merge onto NC 147 North via the ramp on the left toward Durham; follow it 4.9 miles. Take the Duke Street exit, Exit 12C. Turn slightly right onto South Duke Street and follow it 4.3 miles. South Duke Street becomes North Roxboro Street/US 501 North; follow it 0.1 mile until you reach the entrance to West Point on the Eno, and park on the right.

From Durham, take I-40 West for 9 miles. Merge onto NC 147 North via Exit 279B toward Durham/Downtown and follow it 5.7 miles. Take the Briggs Avenue exit, Exit 10, toward Durham Technical Community College and follow it 0.2 mile. Turn left onto South Briggs Avenue and follow it 0.2 mile. Merge onto NC 147 South via the ramp on the left and follow it 2.5 miles. Take the Ellis Road exit, Exit 8. Turn left onto Ellis Road and merge onto NC 147 North via the ramp on the left toward Durham; follow it 4.9 miles. Take the Duke Street exit, Exit 12C. Turn slightly right onto South Duke Street and follow it 4.3 miles. South Duke Street becomes North Roxboro Street/US 501 North; follow it 0.1 mile until you reach the entrance to West Point on the Eno, and park on the right.

Appendix A:
Outdoor Retailers

Raleigh

DICK'S SPORTING GOODS
dickssportinggoods.com
8021 Brier Creek Parkway, #100
Raleigh, NC 27617
919-806-5153

401 Crossroads Blvd.
Cary, NC 27511
919-851-7721

145 Shenstone Blvd.
Garner, NC 27529
919-662-4177

EDDIE BAUER
eddiebauer.com
4325 Glenwood Ave.
Raleigh, NC 27612
919-571-1571

GREAT OUTDOOR PROVISION CO.
greatoutdoorprovision.com
2017 Cameron St.
Raleigh, NC 27605
919-833-1741

RALEIGH RUNNING OUTFITTERS
raleighrunning.com
7449 Six Forks Rd.
Raleigh, NC 27615
919-870-8998

2773 NC 55
Cary, NC 27519
919-362-8282

REI
rei.com
4291 The Circle at North Hills
Raleigh, NC 27609
919-571-5031

1751 Walnut St.
Cary, NC 27511
919-233-8444

TOBACCO ROAD OUTDOORS
tobaccoroadoutdoors.com
225 N. Salem St., #100
Apex, NC 27502
919-267-9353

THE WALKING COMPANY
thewalkingcompany.com
5959 Triangle Town Blvd., #2069
Raleigh, NC 27616
919-792-2433

1105 Walnut St., #1126
Cary, NC 27511
919-467-1294

Durham

DICK'S SPORTING GOODS
dickssportinggoods.com
5422 New Hope Commons Dr.
Durham, NC 27707
919-493-9884

EDDIE BAUER
eddiebauer.com
6910 Fayetteville St.
Durham, NC 27713
919-484-9787

GREAT OUTDOOR PROVISION CO.
greatoutdoorprovision.com
1800 E. Franklin St., #23
Chapel Hill, NC 27514
919-933-6148

REI
rei.com
6911 Fayetteville St., #109
Durham, NC 27713
919-806-3442

Appendix B:
Hiking Clubs

CHAPEL HILL–DURHAM HIKERS
meetup.com/chapel-hill-durham-hikers

DUKE OUTING CLUB
dukegroups.duke.edu/outing

PIEDMONT APPALACHIAN TRAIL HIKERS
path-at.org

PIEDMONT HIKING & OUTING CLUB
piedmonthikingandoutingclub.org

RALEIGH OUTDOOR CLUB
raleighoutdoorclub.org

RALEIGH SKI AND OUTING CLUB
raleighskiandoutingclub.org

TRIANGLE HIKING & OUTDOORS GROUP
meetup.com/adventures

Index

About the Author

Joshua Kinser is a writer and musician based in Chimney Rock, North Carolina. His passion for travel has led him to work at some of the coolest jobs in the world, including not only writing guidebooks and travel articles for magazines and newspapers but also providing musical entertainment on cruise ships and exploring national parks as a backcountry-wildlife biology technician.

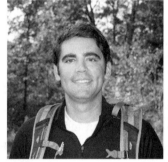

photographed by Jessica Nile

Josh has written several hiking guidebooks to the Southeast, including _Five-Star Trails: Charlotte_ (Menasha Ridge Press, 2012). He is also the author of Moon Handbooks' _Florida Gulf Coast_ guide, along with several comical travel books, including _Following Mowgli: An Appalachian Trail Adventure with the World's Most Hilarious Dog,_ about hiking the southern Appalachian Trail with his destructive but lovable German shepherd. Josh has published more than 200 articles online for websites such as Trails.com, eHow, and USA Today Travel. In addition, he has worked as a staff writer for Gannett's _Pensacola News Journal_ and contributed to such publications as _Sail Magazine, Bonita & Estero Magazine,_ and _Times of the Islands._

As a backcountry-biology tech, he has worked in Florida, Hawaii Volcanoes National Park, Glacier National Park in Montana, and the forestlands surrounding Yosemite National Park in California. Working as a drummer aboard cruise ships, and as a travel writer, has taken him all over the world, including the Caribbean, Australia, China, Japan, and New Zealand.

DEAR CUSTOMERS AND FRIENDS,

SUPPORTING YOUR INTEREST IN OUTDOOR ADVENTURE, travel, and an active lifestyle is central to our operations, from the authors we choose to the locations we detail to the way we design our books. Menasha Ridge Press was incorporated in 1982 by a group of veteran outdoorsmen and professional outfitters. For many years now, we've specialized in creating books that benefit the outdoors enthusiast.

Almost immediately, Menasha Ridge Press earned a reputation for revolutionizing outdoors- and travel-guidebook publishing. For such activities as canoeing, kayaking, hiking, backpacking, and mountain biking, we established new standards of quality that transformed the whole genre, resulting in outdoor-recreation guides of great sophistication and solid content. Menasha Ridge continues to be outdoor publishing's greatest innovator.

The folks at Menasha Ridge Press are as at home on a white-water river or mountain trail as they are editing a manuscript. The books we build for you are the best they can be, because we're responding to your needs. Plus, we use and depend on them ourselves.

We look forward to seeing you on the river or the trail. If you'd like to contact us directly, join in at www.trekalong.com or visit us at www.menasharidge.com. We thank you for your interest in our books and the natural world around us all.

SAFE TRAVELS,

Bob Sehlinger

BOB SEHLINGER
PUBLISHER